Healing with Precision: Integrating Ayurveda and Advanced Laser Techniques for Surgeons

Dr. Praveen Sahave

KORYFI GROUP
of Media & Publications

Healing with Precision: Integrating Ayurveda and Advanced Laser Techniques for Surgeons

Author: Dr. Praveen Sahave

ISBN: 9788198821492

Price: Rs. 1499/-

First Published in June, 2025

Publisher & Printer:

Koryfi Group of Media and Publications
Address: B-515, 5th Floor, Shalin Square, Nr. Lalgebi Circle,
S. P. Ring Road, Hathijan, Ahmedabad, Gujarat, India - 382445
Phone: +91-635 635 60 70 | **Email:** editor@koryfigroup.org
Website: book.koryfigroup.org

Cover Designer:
Nikhil Panchal

Author Biography

Dr. Praveen N. Sahave,
MS (Shalya), FRACS, DIP. Cosmetic Laser Gynaecology
General Surgeon | Ayurveda Consultant | Laser Proctology Specialist

Dr. Praveen N. Sahave is a pioneering figure in the field of integrative surgery, blending the timeless principles of Ayurveda with cutting-edge advancements in laser proctology. With over two decades of clinical, academic, and surgical experience, Dr. Sahave stands at the forefront of modern Ayurvedic surgery, transforming how anorectal disorders are diagnosed, treated, and understood.

A graduate BAMS from SGACGurukunj -Mozari, Amravati and post-graduate MS (ShalyaTantra) from Government Ayurvedic College, Nagpur (MUHS Nashik), Dr. Sahave further honed his expertise with international training in BIEM laser technology from Zhengzhou, China, and advanced proctology from Sri Lankan and Jordanian experts. He holds a Diploma in Cosmetic Gynaecology and a Fellowship in Proctology (FRACS), cementing his position as a leading innovator in minimally invasive surgical techniques.

He is the Founder and Director of Abhyudya Piles & Laser Superspecialty Hospital, Nagpur, India's premier center for laser-based anorectal surgeries. He has trained over 120 surgeons nationally and internationally, including MBBS MS and BAMS MS professionals, and continues to lead monthly training programs for laser and BIEM technologies.

An accomplished academician and Ex-Associate Professor at C.G. Ayurveda College, Rajnandgaon, Dr. Sahave has also served as Secretary of NIMA Proctology, Nagpur. His deep commitment to society is reflected in his extensive charitable work — having conducted over 5,000 free surgeries for underprivileged patients and launching the nationwide "Piles Mukti Abhiyan."

He is president of Punyashlok Ahillyadevi Yuva Manch (Rg.no-286/2023) NGO .Also Vice president of Maharashtra Throw Ball Association .He is social activist.

Dr. Sahave is the recipient of over 36prestigious awards, including:

- BEST AYURVEDA SURGEON OF INDIA AWARD, Delhi
- India Leadership Award2005
- AYURVISHARAD AWARD by Himalaya Drug Company, Bangalore, in 2005.

2017

- Brand Ambassador of Biem Technology in India - 2017 (Zhengzhou, China)
- Samaj Bhushan Award by Dhangar Yuvak Mandal - 2017 (Nagpur)

2018

- Ahilya Ratna Award - 2018 (Pune)
- Best Piles Surgeon of Maharashtra - 2018 (Bangalore)
- ŸYoung Outstanding laser Surgeon of Maharashtra - 2018 (Bangalore)
- National Zero Mile Award - 2018 (Nagpur)
- Times Health Care Achiever Award - 2018 (Mumbai)
- Punyashloka Ahilya Medico Award - 2018 (Pune)
- Mahamitra Puraskar by Hon. C.M. Devendra Fadnavis - 2018 (Mumbai)
- Yuvapratap State Level Krishi-samajik Award – 2018(Pune)
- Buldana Bhushan Award by Buldana Jilha NagrikMandal - 2018 (Nagpur)

2019

- FRACS Fellowship in Proctology - 2019(Bhubaneshwar, Orissa)
- Sakal Excellence Award by Hon. Nitin Gadkari - 2019 (Nagpur)
- Pratigya Social Impact Award for Proctology by Dia Mirza - 2019 (New Delhi)

2020

- Excellence in LASER Proctocology 2020-2021
- India Icon Awards 2021 (Bangalore)
- Leadership Award for Best Piles Laser Hospital of Nagpur – 2021

- Sushrut Award 2021 Extraordinary Work in Proctology (Pune)
- Vaidya Khadiwaale Sushrut Award 2021 (Pune) - 2022
- Dhanavantri Award - 2022 (Hyderabad) - 2023
- Best Laser Piles Surgeon of Nagpur (Big Impact 2023)
- Yashavant Ratna Award - 2023 (Pune)
- Red Pride Awards, Nagpur (RedFM) - 2024

He even started his own YouTube channel named 'Praveen Sahave' which provides guidance and advice on piles. His solid online presence on various platforms like YouTube and Instagram has led to a strong social media following. He has around 171K followers on Instagram and 15k subscribers on YouTube. A lot of people have gained vital information from his channel. Awards and Recognitions Dr. Praveen Sahave has secured 35 National and 1 International Award for his pioneering work at just 42 years old. Skillfully merging Ayurveda and laser technology, he excels in treating hemorrhoids, fissures, and pilonidal sinuses. Trained by Dr. Firaz in Laser Proctology and Ayurvedic Surgery, he leads Nagpur's Punyashlok Ahilyabai Yuva Munch, conducting free medical camps. With 120+ lectures, workshops, and research published in Tokyo's International Journal, Dr. Sahave's impact is truly remarkable. Following are some of the notable awards and recognitions he has received for his exceptional work in the field of healthcare:

Website: www.pilesfistulacure.com

Email: pppsahave@gmail.com

Phone: +91 9326863318 | +91 9970743318

Dedication Note

"कर्तारमपि कार्यस्य समर्थं न प्रयोजकम्।
समयं च प्रवृत्तिं च विनाऽपि फलमज्ञयम।।"

"Even a capable doer (person) cannot accomplish a task alone.
Without the right time and proper initiative, success is uncertain."

To
My beloved parents,
whose unwavering faith, blessings, and sacrifices laid the foundation of my journey.

To
My wife and children,
for their patience, love, and silent strength during every late night of research and service.

To
My teachers and mentors,
for illuminating my path with both ancient wisdom and modern vision.

To
Every patients,
whose healing inspired the evolution of this integrative surgical philosophy.

And to
The future surgeons of the world,
may this book become a guiding light in your pursuit of precision, compassion, and holistic healing.

— Dr. Praveen Sahave, MS (Shalya)

My Inspiration

My Parents

Mr. Narayan Sahave & Mrs. Kusum Sahave

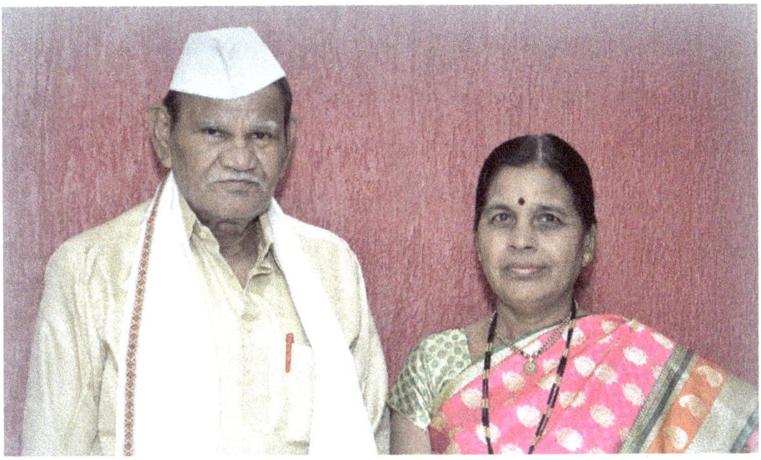

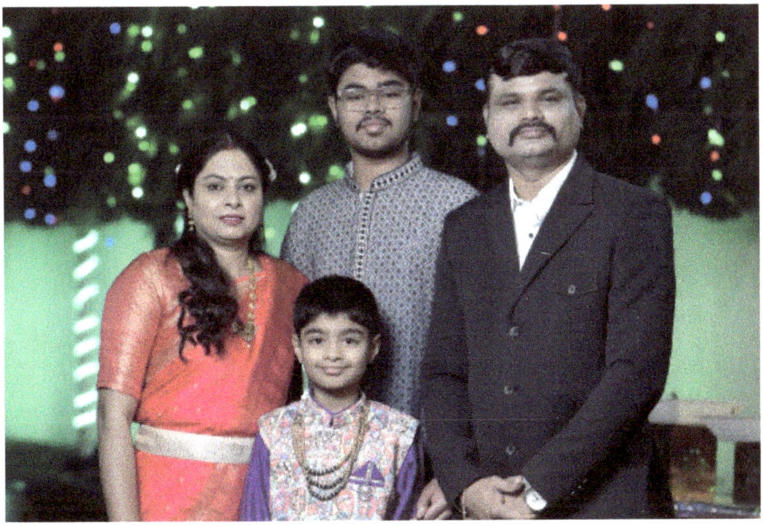

Dr. Puja Sahave | Parth Sahave | Parva Sahave

Table of Content

Part 1:
Foundations of Healing

Ch. 1
Introduction:
The Need for Integrative Surgery

In today's fast-paced medical environment, precision, safety, and faster recovery are the gold standards for any surgical practice. As newer technologies such as laser proctology revolutionize patient care, there is a growing realization that modern methods alone may not address the full spectrum of healing. Pain relief, tissue regeneration, recurrence prevention, and holistic recovery often require something more.

This is where Ayurveda, the ancient Indian system of medicine, holds unmatched value. Ayurveda emphasizes individual constitution (*Prakriti*), disease causation (*Nidana*), and long-term tissue health (*Dhatu Pushti*)—elements that modern surgery sometimes overlooks. It becomes evident that both systems have unique strengths:

Modern laser surgery offers precision and minimal invasiveness. Ayurveda brings in preventive, rehabilitative, and tissue-restorative depth.

This book explores how an integrative surgical model can be developed, where laser precision meets Ayurvedic wisdom to enhance patients outcomes. The intention is not to replace but to blend, creating a dual-powered surgical ecosystem that:

- Respects evidence-based advancements
- Upholds ancient bioethical principles
- Improves overall healing, not just disease eradication

Goals of Integrative Surgery:

- Faster wound healing
- Fewer complications (e.g., infection, fibrosis)
- Recurrence prevention through *Dosha Bala*ncing
- Improved patient satisfaction and long-term outcomes

This model also redefines the surgeon's role: not just a technician of tissues, but a holistic healer guided by the science of life—Ayurveda.

References

1. Dwivedi, G., & Dwivedi, S. (2007). Sushruta – the Clinician – Teacher par Excellence. Indian Journal of Chest Diseases and Allied Sciences.
2. Sharma, P.V. (2001). Shalya Tantra (Sushruta Samhita). Chaukhambha Visvabharati.
3. Rao, R. (2015). Integrative Approaches in Proctology. Journal of Ayurveda & Integrative Medicine.

Ch. 2
Understanding Ayurveda: A Timeless Science

Introduction

Ayurveda, derived from "Ayuh" (life) and "Veda" (knowledge), is the ancient Indian system of medicine. More than just a medical tradition, it is a comprehensive life science that promotes Balance in body (*Sharira*), mind (*Manas*), and spirit (*Atma*).

1. Definition of Ayurveda

Charaka Samhita – Sutra*Sthana* 1.41:

हिताहितं सुखं दुःखमायुस्तस्य हिताहितम्।
मानं च तच्च यत्रोक्तमायुर्वेदः स उच्यते।।

Transliteration:

Hitāhitam sukham duhkham āyus tasya hitāhitam |
Mānam ca tacca yatroktam āyurvedah sa ucyate ||

Translation:

Ayurveda is that science which describes what is good and bad for life, the happy and unhappy life, its promotive and non-promotive aspects, and the measure of life itself.

Context:

This verse defines the scope of Ayurveda as a guide to the ideal way of living, not merely treating diseases.

2. The Tridosha Theory

Sushruta Samhita – Sutra*Sthana* 21.8:

वायुपित्तकफाश्चैते त्रयः दोषाः समास्तदा।
समाः स्वास्थ्यमनुयान्ति विकृता विकृतिं गताः।।

Transliteration:

Vāyu-pitta-kaphāś caite trayaḥ doṣāḥ samās tadā |
Samāḥ svāsthyaṁ anuyānti vikṛtā vikṛtiṁ gatāḥ ||

Translation:

Vata, *Pitta*, and *Kapha* are the three *Dosha*s. When in Balance, they sustain health; when imbalanced, they lead to disease.

Context:

This is foundational to Ayurveda's diagnostic and therapeutic approach—health is harmony among *Dosha*s.

3. Preventive over Curative

Ashtanga Hridaya – Sutra*Sthana* 1.20:

न रोगाः शाश्वतं कंचिद्रोगिणं नोपतिष्ठिरे।
युक्तिकृत्यं प्रशंसन्ति न केवलं भिषग्जनाः।।

Transliteration:

Na rogāḥ śāśvataṁ kaṁcid rogiṇaṁ nopatiṣṭhire |
Yuktikṛtyaṁ praśaṁsanti na kevalaṁ bhiṣagjanāḥ ||

Translation:

Diseases do not affect a person forever. Wise actions (proper regimen) are praised not only by physicians but by all.

Context:

Ayurveda emphasizes "*Swasthasya Swasthya rakshanam*"—preserving health—before attempting to treat illness.

4. Purpose of Ayurveda

Charaka Samhita – Sutra*Sthana* 30.26:

धर्मार्थकाममोक्षाणामारोग्यं मूलमुत्तमम् ।
रोगास्तस्यापहर्तारः श्रेयसो जीवनस्य च ।।

Transliteration:

Dharmārtha-kāma-mokṣāṇām ārogyaṁ mūlam uttamam |
Rogās tasyāpahartāraḥ śreyaso jīvanasya ca ||

Translation:

Health is the supreme foundation of virtue, wealth, desire, and liberation. Diseases destroy both health and life's purpose.

Context:

Ayurveda supports not just survival, but fulfillment of the four Purusharthas—the goals of life.

5. Holistic Approach

Ashtanga Hridaya – Sutra*Sthana* 1.2:

शरीरेंद्रियसत्त्वात्मसंयोगो धर्मार्थकाममोक्षाणाम् उपायः ।

Transliteration:

Śarīrendriya-sattvātma-saṁyogo dharmārtha-kāma-mokṣāṇām upāyaḥ.

Translation:

The union of body, senses, mind, and soul is the means to achieve virtue, wealth, desire, and liberation.

Context:

Ayurveda treats the whole person, integrating physical, mental, and spiritual dimensions.

Conclusion

Ayurveda is not merely a system of medicine but a blueprint for balanced living. Rooted in timeless wisdom and guided by deep philosophical insight, it remains relevant today as a science of life and art of healing.

6. Dinacharya (Daily Routine)

Ashtanga Hridaya – Sutra*Sthana* 2.1:

बुद्धिः स्वस्थेन्द्रियार्थेषु धर्मार्थकाममोक्षदा ।
हिता हितं सुखं दुःखं आयुस्तस्य हिताहितम् ।।

Transliteration:

Buddhiḥ svasthendriyārtheṣu dharmārthakāmamokṣadā |
Hitāhitaṁ sukhaṁ duḥkhaṁ āyus tasya hitāhitam ||

Translation:

A balance intellect concerning the objects of the senses helps achieve the goals of life (virtue, wealth, desire, and liberation). What is wholesome and unwholesome, pleasant and painful, and beneficial or harmful to life must be understood.

Context:

Daily discipline cultivates clarity, balance, and longevity.

7. Ritucharya (Seasonal Regimen)

Charaka Samhita – Sutra*Sthana* 6.3:

ऋतुभिः कालजातेन देशेनात्मबलाबलम् ।
वयसा व्याधितश्चैव बुद्ध्वा रोगं विनिर्णयेत् ।।

Transliteration:

Ṛtubhiḥ kālajātena deśenātmabalābalam |
Vayasā vyādhitaś caiva buddhvā rogaṁ vinirṇayet ||

Translation:
In diagnosis, one must consider the impact of seasons, time, locality, body strength, age, and disease nature.

Context:
Ayurveda's adaptability lies in adjusting lifestyle and diet with the seasons to maintain *doshic* balance.

8. Ahara (Wholesome Diet)

Charaka Samhita – Sutrasthana 28.45:

मात्राशी नात्यशीतोष्णं नातिद्रुतमथापि वा।
नातिमन्दं न चाऽत्युष्णं नात्यग्रं च प्रवर्तयेत्।।

Transliteration:
Mātrāśī nātyaśītoṣṇaṁ nātidrutamathāpi vā |
Nāti mandaṁ na cā'tyuṣṇaṁ nātyagraṁ ca pravartayet ||

Translation:
Food should be consumed in proper quantity—not too hot, too cold, too fast, too slow, nor too spicy or bland.

Context:
Ayurveda stresses mindful eating for digestion (*Agni*) and vitality.

9. Rasayana (Rejuvenation Therapy)

Charaka Samhita – Chikitsa Sthana 1.1.7:

आयुः प्रज्ञा स्मृतिर्वर्णो बलं ओजोऽग्निरेव च।
रसायनानां प्रधानं हि फलं स्वास्थ्यं च शाश्वतम्।।

Transliteration:
Āyuḥ prajñā smṛtir varṇo balaṁ ojo'gnir eva ca |
Rasāyanānāṁ pradhānaṁ hi phalaṁ svāsthyaṁ ca śāśvatam ||

Translation:

The prime benefits of *Rasayana* (rejuvenation) are long life, intelligence, memory, complexion, strength, vitality, and everlasting health.

Context:

Rasayana is more than medicine; it's the science of anti-aging and inner vitality.

10. Shalya (Surgical Science)

Sushruta Samhita – Sutrasthana 1.14:

शस्त्रं श्रेयो बलवद्भिश्च यत्र व्याधिः प्रशाम्यति।
तत्र भैषज्यमर्थं च न च मूढेन सेवितम्।।

Transliteration:

Śastraṁ śreyo balavadbhiś ca yatra vyādhiḥ praśāmyati |
Tatra bhaiṣajyam arthaṁ ca na ca mūḍhena sevitam ||

Translation:

Surgery is superior where the disease is not cured by medicine alone. But it should only be used wisely—not by the ignorant.

Context:

Sushruta, the father of surgery, emphasized surgical precision, ethics, and competence.

11. Mind and Consciousness

Charaka Samhita – Sharira *Sthana* 1.137:

मनः स्रोतसि सञ्जातं, जीवितं चेतनालयः।
येन बुद्धिः स्मृतिः प्रज्ञा मनः कर्मेन्द्रियैः सह।।

Transliteration:

Manaḥ srotasi sañjātaṁ, jīvitaṁ cetanālayaḥ |
Yena buddhiḥ smṛtiḥ prajñā manaḥ karmendriyaiḥ saha ||

Translation:
The mind resides in a subtle channel; it is the abode of consciousness, enabling intelligence, memory, and perception along with sensory organs.

Context:
Ayurveda recognizes the mind-body-spirit continuum central to all healing.

Ayurveda, the ancient Indian science of life and healing, is not just a medical system—it is a way of understanding life, health, and the universe. Derived from two Sanskrit words—"Ayuh" (life) and "Veda" (knowledge)—Ayurveda provides a holistic approach to health and disease management, rooted in natural law and centuries of practical experience.

Origins and Philosophical Foundation
Ayurveda dates back more than 5,000 years, documented in texts like the *Charaka Samhita*, *Sushruta Samhita*, and *Ashtanga Hridaya*m. It is based on *Panchamahabhuta Siddhanta*—the theory of five elements:

1. *Prithvi* (Earth)
2. *Apas* (Water)
3. *Tejas* (Fire)
4. *Vayu* (Air)
5. *Akasha* (Space)

These elements combine to form the *Tridosha*s—*Vata*, *Pitta*, and *Kapha*—which govern all physiological and psychological processes in the body.

***Tridosha* Theory and Its Surgical Relevance**
- *Vata Dosha* governs motion and nerve impulses; it must

be controlled during and after surgery to avoid spasms, constipation, and anxiety.
- *Pitta Dosha* governs metabolism and inflammation—key in wound healing and infection.
- *Kapha Dosha* governs structure and fluid balance; its im*Bala*nce can lead to delayed healing or fibrosis.

In the surgical context, balancing *Dosha*s before, during, and after an operation ensures better tissue response, faster wound healing, and less postoperative morbidity.

Ayurveda as a Clinical Science

Far from being mystical or outdated, Ayurveda uses detailed diagnostic tools such as:

1. *Nadi Pariksha* (pulse diagnosis)
2. *Mala-Mutra Pariksha* (stool and urine analysis)
3. *Jihva Pariksha* (tongue examination)
4. *Prakriti* Analysis (body constitution assessment)

These enable personalized treatment protocols that modern systems now aspire to replicate through genomics and personalized medicine.

Surgical Depth in Ayurveda

Ayurveda is also a surgical science, as seen in:

1. *Kaychikitsa* (medicine)
2. *Balrog* (Paedeatric)
3. *Grahdosh* (Psychology)
4. *Shalakya Tantra* (ENT & ophthalmology)
5. *Shalya Tantra* (surgery)
6. *Agad Tantra* (Toxicology)
7. *Vajikaran* (Rejuvanation)

1. Kayachikitsa (Internal Medicine / Therapeutics)

Charaka Samhita – Chikitsa Sthana 15.5:

कायशुद्धिः प्रधानं हि चिकित्सायाः प्रयोजनम्।
सर्वेषां रोगणां हन्ता तद्वत् कायचिकित्सितम्।।

Transliteration:

Kāyaśuddhiḥ pradhānaṁ hi cikitsāyāḥ prayojanam |
Sarveṣāṁ rogaṇāṁ hantā tadvat kāyacikitsitam ||

Translation:

Purification of the body is the primary goal of treatment. Internal medicine eliminates the root causes of all diseases.

Context:

Kayachikitsa deals with systemic disorders and the correction of doshic imbalances through diet, herbs, and lifestyle.

2. Kaumarabhritya / Balaroga (Pediatrics)

Ashtanga Hridaya – Uttara Tantra 1.5:

बालस्य हि शरीरं स्यात् स्नेहेन परिवर्धितम्।
शीतातपविपर्यासे क्षिप्रं विकृतिमृच्छति।।

Transliteration:

Bālasya hi śarīraṁ syāt snehena parivardhitam |
Śītātapaviparyāse kṣipraṁ vikṛtim ṛcchati ||

Translation:

The child's body, developed with nourishment and care, is delicate and quickly disturbed by cold, heat, and external factors.

Context:

Kaumarabhritya focuses on growth, immunity, and developmental care from infancy to adolescence.

3. **Graha Roga (Psychology & Psychiatry)**

Charaka Samhita – Nidana Sthana 7.4:

राजयक्ष्मा भगन्दरशोऽर्बुदग्रन्थिशर्कराः ।
मानसाः सप्त रोगाश्च दैवोपहतचेतसाम् ।।

Transliteration:

Rājayakṣmā bhagandaraśo'rbuda-granthi-śarkarāḥ |
Mānasāḥ sapta rogāś ca daivopahata-cetasām ||

Translation:

Diseases like tuberculosis, fistula, tumors, stones, and seven types of mental disorders arise in those whose minds are afflicted by unseen (*daivika*) causes.

Context:

Graha Dosha denotes psychological or psychiatric disturbances, explained through both metaphysical and neurobehavioral lenses.

4. **Shalakya Tantra (ENT and Ophthalmology)**

Sushruta Samhita – Uttara Tantra 1.5:

शिरसोऽङ्गेषु सर्वेषु प्रधानत्वात् प्रधानतः ।
शिरोधार्याण्युपक्रान्ता नेत्रकर्णादिनाशनात् ।।

Transliteration:

Śiraso'ṅgeṣu sarveṣu pradhānatvāt pradhānataḥ |
Śirodhāryāṇy upakrāntā netra-karṇādi-nāśanāt ||

Translation:

Among all organs, the head is the most vital; thus, diseases affecting the eyes, ears, nose, and mouth must be treated with great care.

Context:

Shalakya Tantra is Ayurveda's specialist field dealing with diseases of the eyes (*Netra*), ears (*karna*), nose (*nasa*), and throat (*mukha/gala*).

5. Shalya Tantra (Surgery)

Sushruta Samhita – Sutra*Sthana* 1.8:

येन विज्ञानशस्त्रार्थं शल्यं साक्षात्कृतं पुनः ।
स च शास्त्रार्थतत्त्वज्ञः स भवेद्योग्यतत्त्ववित् ।।

Transliteration:

Yena vijñānaśastrārthaṁ śalyaṁ sākṣātkṛtaṁ punaḥ |
Sa ca śāstrārthatattvajñaḥ sa bhaved yogyatattvavit ||

Translation:

He who knows both the science and art of surgery, and understands the essence of the texts, is a truly competent surgeon.

Context:

Sushruta emphasized hands-on training, ethics, and intellectual precision in surgical practice.

6. Agada Tantra (Toxicology)

Charaka Samhita – Sutrasthana 23.4:

सर्वेषां विषविज्ञानं नित्यमेव विवेकिना ।
अगदार्थं भिषग्भिश्च विज्ञेयं नित्ययत्नतः ।।

Transliteration:

Sarveṣāṁ viṣa-vijñānaṁ nityam eva vivekinā |
Agadārthaṁ bhiṣagbhis ca vijñeyaṁ nityayatnataḥ ||

Translation:

A wise physician must always be well-versed in toxicology (*visha-vidya*) for proper antidotal therapy (*Agada*).

Context:

Agad Tantra deals with poisoning, insect bites, snake venom, and contaminated food, a crucial branch of Ayurvedic emergency care.

7. Vajikarana (Aphrodisiac / Rejuvenation / Fertility)

Charaka Samhita – Chikitsa Sthana 2.1.3:

वाजी स्यान्नाम यः स्त्रीषु रमते न पराजयेत्।
तस्माद्वाजीकरणमेतभ्द्वति सन्ततौ हितम्।।

Transliteration:

Vājī syān nāma yaḥ strīṣu ramate na parājayet |
Tasmād vājīkaraṇam etad bhavati santatau hitam ||

Translation:

He is called "*Vaji*" who can enjoy conjugal life without fatigue or failure; hence, *Vajikarana* is beneficial for vitality and progeny.

Context:

Vajikarana promotes sexual health, reproductive vitality, and hormonal rejuvenation, especially important in *Rasayana* context.

The *Sushruta Samhita*, considered the world's earliest surgical manual, describes:

- Over 300 surgical procedures
- 120+ surgical instruments
- Dissection techniques
- Advanced operations like rhinoplasty, lithotripsy, and even fracture management

1. Acharya Sushruta documented over 300 surgeries, including those for:

Vrana (wounds), *Arsha* (piles), *Bhagandara* (fistula)

Netra roga (eye diseases), *Nasa Sandhana* (rhinoplasty)

Ashmari (bladder stone), *Bhagna* (fractures)

शस्त्रकर्माणि सर्वाणि यानि यानि प्रकीर्तितम्।
तानि सर्वाणि विज्ञेयं सदा योग्येन सत्वता।।

(Sushruta Samhita, Sutra Sthana 1.8)

Transliteration:
Śastrakarmāṇi sarvāṇi yāni yāni prakīrtitam |
Tāni sarvāṇi vijñeyaṁ sadā yogyena satvatā ||

Meaning:
All the various surgical operations described should be thoroughly understood and performed only by one who is skilled and courageous.

2. 120+ Surgical Instruments (शस्त्र–यन्त्र)

Sushruta describes 101 blunt instruments (*Yantras*) and 20 sharp instruments (*Shastras*), including:

Mandalagra (circular knife), *Karapatra* (saw), *Vrihhipatra* (scalpel), *Shalaka* (probe)

शस्त्रं शतं चैकं दश चैव यन्त्राणि चैकविंशतिः।
समासेनोच्यते संख्या शस्त्रयन्त्राणि भारत।।

(Sushruta Samhita, Sutra Sthana 7.3)

Transliteration:
Śastraṁ śataṁ caikaṁ daśa caiva yantrāṇi caikaviṁśatiḥ |
Samāsenocyate saṁkhyā śastrayāntrāṇi bhārata ||

Meaning:
There are 101 sharp instruments and 20 blunt instruments (total 121) used in surgery.

3. Dissection Techniques (मृतशरीर विच्छेदन)

Sushruta was the first in the world to advocate cadaver dissection to study anatomy.

(Sushruta Samhita, Sharira Sthana 5.46)

स्थूलपेशिशिरापर्वणि युक्ते च मृतशरीरे ।
तं सप्तरात्रमुदके स्थापयित्वा विमृज्य च ।।

Transliteration:

Sthūlapeśiśirāparvaṇi yukte ca mṛtaśarīre |
Taṁ saptarātramudake sthāpayitvā vimṛjya ca ||

Meaning:

A body with properly developed muscles and joints should be kept in water for seven days and then gently scraped to study the anatomy.

4. Rhinoplasty (नासासन्धान)

*Sushruta's nasa*l reconstruction technique is the earliest known form of plastic surgery.

(Sushruta Samhita, Chikitsa Sthana 16.27)

चर्मणि गृह्यते यत्नात् कपोलात्त्वग्विशेषतः ।
तं सम्यग्व्यधिविष्टार्य स्थाने स्थाप्य प्रणामयेत् ।।

Transliteration:

Carmaṇi gṛhyate yatnāt kapolāttvagviśeṣataḥ |
Taṁ samyagvyadhiviṣṭārya sthāne sthāpya praṇāmayet ||

Meaning:

A special type of skin (flap) should be carefully taken from the cheek and attached to the damaged part of the nose to reconstruct it.

5. Lithotripsy (अश्मरिभेदनम)

Sushruta describes the removal of urinary stones via perineal incision.

Sanskrit Shloka (Sushruta Samhita, Chikitsa Sthana 7.10)

पार्श्ववस्थे यत्नतः क्षेत्रे सम्यक् चेदयेत् त्वचम्।
मांसं चान्तरमाकृष्य शोणितं सम्यगुद्धरेत्।।

Transliteration:

Pārśvavasthe yatnataḥ kṣetre samyak cedayet tvacam |
Māṁsaṁ cāntaramākṛṣya śoṇitaṁ samyaguddharet ||

Meaning:

Position the patient properly, carefully incise the skin and muscle, and remove the stone from the bladder by pulling it out.

6. Fracture & Dislocation Management (भङ्ग, सन्धिमुक्त)

Sushruta identified 12 types of fractures and 6 types of dislocations, and prescribed traction, bandaging, splints, and herbal healing.

(Sushruta Samhita, Chikitsa Sthana 3.28)

भङ्गे भिषग्बन्धनं कुर्यात् स्नेहस्वेदपुरःसरम्।
स्थानं चापि समासाद्य स्वाभाविकमपाक्रमे।।

Transliteration:

Bhaṅge bhiṣagbandhanaṁ kuryāt snehasvedapuraḥsaram |
Sthānaṁ cāpi samāsādya svābhāvikamapākrame ||

Meaning:

In case of fractures, after administering oil and fomentation, the physician should align the bone and apply splints and bandages to immobilize and heal.

Conclusion: Ancient Surgical Mastery

Aspect	Detail	Sanskrit Reference
Surgical Instruments	121 types	S.S. *Sutra* 7.3
Dissection	Cadaver study	S.S. *Sharira* 5.46
Rhinoplasty	Nasal repair	S.S. *Chikitsa* 16.27
Lithotomy	Stone removal	S.S. *Chikitsa* 7.10
Fracture care	Bone healing	S.S. *Chikitsa* 3.28

This foundational surgical knowledge integrates surprisingly well with modern minimally invasive techniques such as laser proctology and other surgical procedures.

Integrative Potential

Modern studies have validated Ayurvedic herbs and practices:

Ayurvedic Herbs in Post-Operative & Surgical Care

1. Curcuma longa (Haridra – Turmeric)

Actions:

- *Shotha-hara* (anti-inflammatory)
- *Krimighna* (anti-microbial)
- *Raktashodhaka* (blood purifier)
- *Vranashodhaka* & *Vranaropaka* (wound cleaning and healing)

Modern Correlation:

Curcumin is a potent anti-inflammatory, anti-bacterial, and antioxidant.

Aids in preventing post-op infections and accelerating healing.

(*Bhavaprakasha* Reference):

हरिद्रा त्वग्रुजा कण्ठ्या कृमिघ्नी श्लेष्मनाशिनी।
व्रणमेहकुष्ठहरिणी दीपन्या रचनासु च।।

Transliteration:
Haridrā tvagrujā kaṇṭhyā krimighnī śleṣmanāśinī |
Vraṇameha-kuṣṭhahariṇī dīpanyā racanāsu ca ||

Meaning:
Haridra (turmeric) is beneficial for skin diseases, worms, *Kapha*-related disorders, wounds, diabetes, and digestive issues.

2. Guggulu (Commiphora mukul)

Actions:

- *Vranaropaka* (wound healer)
- *Lekhana* (scraping action – reduces swelling/fat)
- *Shothahara* (anti-inflammatory)
- Antiseptic and astringent properties

Modern Correlation:
Contains guggulsterones, known to modulate inflammation and accelerate collagen synthesis and tissue repair.

Often used in post-operative herbal formulations like *Kanchanara Guggulu* or *Yograj Guggulu*.

गुग्गुलुस्तिक्तको वर्ण्यः कटुको दीपनो लघुः ।
मेहकुष्ठकफासृग्दोषव्रणशोथार्शसां जयेत् ।।

(Charaka Samhita, Sutra Sthana 4.14)

Transliteration:
Guggulustiktako varṇyaḥ kaṭuko dīpano laghuḥ |
Mehakuṣṭhakaphāsṛgdoṣavraṇaśothārśasāṁ jayet ||

Meaning:
Guggulu is bitter, light, sharp, and beneficial for wounds, swelling, hemorrhoids, *Kapha*, skin diseases, and urinary issues.

3. Triphala (Haritaki, Bibhitaki, Amalaki)

Actions:

- *Amapachana* (digests toxins)
- *Anulomana* (mild laxative for gut clearance)
- *Rasayana* (rejuvenator)
- Supports gut microbiota post-antibiotic or surgical stress

Modern Correlation:
Rich in polyphenols and vitamin C.

Enhances gut health, immunity, and helps with post-op constipation or sluggish metabolism

(*Charaka Samhita*, *Chikitsa Sthana* 1.3.41)

त्रिफला हित्वा दोषान् बलं वर्णं च धारयेत्।
रसायनं च चक्षुष्यं विशेषात् कफपित्तजित्।।

Transliteration:
Triphalā hitvā doṣān balaṁ varṇaṁ ca dhārayet |
Rasāyanaṁ ca cakṣuṣyaṁ viśeṣāt kaphapittajit ||

Meaning:
Triphala balances *Dosha*s, improves strength and complexion, is rejuvenating and especially beneficial for eye and *Pitta-Kapha* disorders.

4. Ashwagandha (Withania somnifera)

Actions:

- *Balya* (strengthens)
- *Rasayana* (rejuvenator)
- *Medhya* (enhances mental clarity)
- *Manovaha-srotas poshana* (nourishes psychological pathways)

Modern Correlation:
Contains withanolides, proven to reduce cortisol and enhance

recovery from surgical stress, trauma, and fatigue.

Excellent adaptogen used in post-op fatigue or debility.

अश्वगन्धा बल्या पुष्टि मेध्यया वृष्यया स्थिरा।
रसायनी च शक्तिघ्नी श्वासकासप्रशामिनी।।

(*Bhavaprakasha* Nighantu)

Transliteration:
Aśvagandhā balyā puṣṭi medhyayā vṛṣyayā sthirā |
Rasāyanī ca śaktighnī śvāsakāsapraśāminī ||

Meaning:
Ashwagandha provides strength, nourishment, intelligence, virility, stability, and relieves respiratory disorders and stress.

Integted Post-Surgical Care – Ayurvedic Approach

Herb	Key Benefit	Modern Use
Haridra (Turmeric)	Antiseptic, wound healer	Topical + oral for healing, anti-infective
Guggulu	Granulation and healing	Internal use for post-op tissue repair
Triphala	Detox, gut motility	Recovery of digestion, antioxidant
Ashwagandha	Anti-stress, immunity builder	Restores energy, modulates cortisol

These can reduce reliance on antibiotics, improve tissue response, and shorten recovery time in surgical patients.

Ayurveda: A Living Science

Ayurveda is not a fossilized tradition—it evolves:

- Incorporates modern tools for diagnosis
- Encourages interdisciplinary collaboration
- Supports evidence-based validation

Modern Integration of Ayurveda

1. Incorporates Modern Tools for Diagnosis

Ayurveda today complements its traditional diagnostic methods like *Nadi Pariksha*, *Jihva Pariksha*, *Mutra–Mala–Netra Pariksha* with modern technologies such as:

- Blood tests, imaging (MRI, CT scan, ultrasound) for internal assessments
- Genetic and metabolic profiling to personalize Ayurvedic protocols (Ayurgenomics)
- Digital *Nadi* devices and AI-based diagnostic platforms enhance pulse reading and *Dosha* evaluation

Ayurvedic Principle + Modern Tool = Precision Diagnosis

2. Encourages Interdisciplinary Collaboration

Modern Ayurveda promotes collaboration with conventional medicine and other systems (homeopathy, naturopathy, allopathy), especially in areas like:

- Psychiatry: Ayurveda + psychotherapy for anxiety, insomnia
- Orthopedics: *Bhagna chikitsa* + physiotherapy
- Oncology: *Rasayana* + chemo/radiotherapy for supportive care
- Cardiology & endocrinology: Integration in managing diabetes, hypertension, thyroid disorders

"Ayurveda doesn't reject modern science – it expands it."

3. Supports Evidence-Based Validation

Ayurveda is increasingly supported by clinical research and peer-reviewed studies:

- Randomized Controlled Trials (RCTs) on herbs like *Ashwagandha*, *Triphala*, and *Brahmi*
- Pharmacological studies validate *Rasayana* drugs' antioxidant, immunomodulatory, and neuroprotective effects
- Government initiatives (e.g., Ministry of AYUSH, CCRAS) funding large-scale clinical trials
- Ayurveda research is now visible in databases like PubMed, Scopus, and Cochrane

Example:

A 2022 RCT published in J-AIM (Journal of Ayurveda and Integrative Medicine) demonstrated Triphala's efficacy in IBS compared to standard allopathic treatment.

Conclusion: Ayurveda in the 21st Century

Principle	Modern Integration
Roga–Rogi Pariksha (Diagnosis)	Imaging, blood tests, genomics
Chikitsa Sutra (Therapy protocols)	Combined with surgery, pharmacotherapy
Rasayana & *Vajikarana*	Studied for anti-aging, stress, fertility
Research-backed usage	Clinical trials, evidence-based protocols
Holistic health	Lifestyle, diet, yoga + modern interventions

By embedding Ayurvedic diagnostics and recovery methods into laser-assisted surgery, we unlock a healing system rooted in nature, precision, and personalization.

References

1. Sharma, R. K., & Dash, B. (1999). Caraka Samhita. Chowkhamba Sanskrit Series Office.
2. Sushruta, Kunjalal Bhishagratna (1907). The Sushruta Samhita. Calcutta.
3. Patwardhan, B. et al. (2005). Ayurveda and traditional Chinese medicine: A comparative overview. eCAM.
4. Tillu, G., Patwardhan, B., & Vaidya, A. D. B. (2012). AYUSH for COVID-19 management. Journal of Ayurveda and Integrative Medicine.

Ch. 3
Modern Surgical Techniques: A Rapid Evolution

Surgery has evolved tremendously over the past century, driven by advances in technology, understanding of human anatomy, and patient care standards. What once were crude and risky interventions have become precise, minimally invasive and patient-centered procedures.

The Journey of Surgical Progress

Ancient Beginnings: Early surgical efforts, including those in Ayurveda (*Sushruta Samhita*) and Hippocratic practices, laid the foundation for understanding anatomy and asepsis.

19th Century Breakthroughs: Introduction of anesthesia and antisepsis revolutionized surgery, drastically reducing pain and infection.

20th Century Advances: Development of antibiotics, blood transfusions, and imaging technologies further improved surgical safety and outcomes.

Minimally Invasive Surgery (MIS)

One of the most transformative leaps has been the rise of minimally invasive techniques, including:

- Laparoscopy: Small incisions with cameras and instruments allowing abdominal surgeries with less trauma.
- Endoscopy: Visualization and intervention within hollow organs.
- Robotic Surgery: Enhances precision and dexterity with computer-assisted tools.

These methods offer:

- Reduced postoperative pain
- Shorter hospital stays
- Faster return to daily activities
- Decreased risk of infection and scarring

Laser Surgery: The New Frontier

Laser technology represents a significant innovation for precision tissue management. Lasers provide:

- High accuracy: Laser beams can target diseased tissue without affecting adjacent healthy tissue.
- Hemostasis: Simultaneous cutting and coagulation reduce bleeding.
- Minimal invasiveness: Ideal for sensitive regions like the anorectal area.
- Less postoperative pain and swelling.

Laser proctology has emerged as a leading technique in managing hemorrhoids, fissures, and *fistulas* with excellent patient satisfaction.

Advances in Imaging and Navigation

Modern surgeons utilize real-time imaging (ultrasound, MRI, CT scans) and navigation systems to:

- Visualize surgical fields in 3D
- Avoid critical structures
- Tailor surgical plans dynamically

This has improved accuracy in complex surgeries, including oncology and reconstructive procedures.

Multidisciplinary Collaboration

Contemporary surgery is no longer the realm of the alone surgeon but a collaborative discipline involving anesthetists, radiologists, pathologists, physiotherapists, and nutritionists. The integration of diverse expertise ensures holistic care and improved outcomes.

Personalized Surgery: The Future

The future of surgery is shifting towards personalized, precision medicine, where genetic, molecular, and physiological patient data inform surgical decisions. This resonates with Ayurvedic principles of individual constitution and personalized treatment, opening the door to integrative surgical models.

References

1. Gawande, A. (2010). Complications: A Surgeon's Notes on an Imperfect Science. Picador.
2. Sharda, R. (2017). Minimally Invasive Surgery: An Overview. Journal of Minimal Access Surgery.
3. Mukherjee, S., & Patra, A. (2021). Laser in anorectal surgery: A comprehensive review. International Journal of Surgery.
4. Smith, R. A., et al. (2019). Personalized surgery and the future of medicine. Journal of Surgical Research.

Ch. 4
Bridging Ancient Wisdom and Modern Innovation

In the realm of healthcare, the quest for healing has often been portrayed as a dichotomy—traditional versus modern, ancient versus contemporary. However, true progress arises not from choosing one over the other, but from harmonizing the best elements of both. This chapter explores the synthesis of Ayurvedic wisdom and modern surgical innovation, focusing on how this integrative approach can transform patient care.

The Complementary Strengths

- Ayurveda's Strengths:
  - Holistic understanding of the human body as a system
  - Emphasis on balance and prevention (*Dosha*s, *Dhatu*s, *Mala*s)
  - Personalized treatment strategies based on *Prakriti*
  - Use of natural remedies and therapies (herbs, *Panchakarma*, *Ksharasutra*)
  - Deep knowledge of wound healing and tissue regeneration

- Modern Surgery's Strengths:
  - High precision, minimally invasive techniques
  - Advanced diagnostic and imaging tools
  - Evidence-based protocols and rapid intervention
  - Innovations like lasers, robotics, and improved anesthesia
  - Standardized sterilization and infection control

Bridging these strengths offers a powerful synergy—the precision and speed of modern technology combined with the holistic, patient-centered philosophy of Ayurveda.

Integrative Surgical Protocols

- Preoperative Phase:

Incorporating Ayurvedic *Prakriti* analysis alongside modern diagnostics (blood tests, imaging) to tailor surgical planning. *Panchakarma* therapies may be used to detoxify and strengthen the patient pre-surgery.

- Intraoperative Phase:

Employing laser and minimally invasive techniques that align with Ayurvedic principles of minimizing tissue trauma and preserving vital energy (*Ojas*). Using Ayurvedic oils and antiseptics to support tissue integrity.

- Postoperative Phase:

Utilizing *Rasayana* therapies, herbal formulations, and dietary regimens to accelerate healing, modulate inflammation, and restore balance. Monitoring *Dosha* status to prevent complications and recurrence.

Case for Integrative Proctology:

Anorectal diseases such as hemorrhoids and *fistulas* are traditionally treated with painful surgical methods that often lead to prolonged recovery and recurrence. Modern laser techniques reduce trauma but sometimes lack holistic patient care. Ayurvedic treatments like *Ksharasutra* therapy have proven effective but can be prolonged and painful.

An integrative approach combining laser precision with Ayurvedic wound care and diet can reduce pain, speed recovery, and lower recurrence rates—offering a model for other surgical disciplines.

Challenges and Solutions

- Knowledge Gap: Bridging the gap between Ayurveda and modern medical practitioners through interdisciplinary training.
- Research Evidence: Conducting rigorous clinical trials to validate integrative protocols.
- Patient Awareness: Educating patients about benefits and safety of combined therapies.
- Regulatory Framework: Developing guidelines for integrative surgical practice.

Future Directions

- Development of integrative surgical centers with multidisciplinary teams.
- Use of digital health tools to monitor Ayurveda parameters alongside modern vitals.
- Expansion of integrative curricula in medical education.
- Collaborative research to establish standardized treatment algorithms.

References

1. Vaidya, A.D.B., & Devasagayam, T.P.A. (2007). Current status of herbal drugs in Ayurveda. Regulatory Toxicology and Pharmacology.
2. Patwardhan, B., & Sharma, P.V. (2008). Integrative approaches to health care: Ayurvedic and Western medicine. Journal of Ayurveda and Integrative Medicine
3. Singh, R.H. (2012). The integration of Ayurveda and modern medicine. Ayurveda Journal
4. Bhatia, S. C. (2016). Integrative medicine in surgical practice: Opportunities and challenges. Indian Journal of Surgery.

Ch. 5
Shalya Tantra:
The Ayurvedic Surgical System

Shalya Tantra, often regarded as the surgical branch of Ayurveda, is a sophisticated and ancient system of surgical knowledge and practice, dating back over 2,500 years. It is one of the eight major branches (*Ashtanga* Ayurveda) and deals extensively with the diagnosis and management of surgical diseases, including trauma, wounds, fractures, and various internal disorders.

Historical Context and Importance

The foundational text for *Shalya Tantra* is the *Sushruta Samhita*, attributed to Sage *Sushruta*, who is considered the "Father of Surgery." This text is a pioneering surgical manual detailing surgical instruments, procedures, and principles that are surprisingly advanced even by today's standards.

Sushruta's contributions include:

- Detailed anatomical descriptions
- Innovative surgical instruments
- Procedures like rhinoplasty, cataract surgery, and fracture management
- Emphasis on aseptic technique and postoperative care

Core Principles of Shalya Tantra

1. *Nidana* (Diagnosis): Detailed understanding of disease causation, including external and internal factors.
2. *Shodhana* (Purification): Preoperative cleansing and detoxification through *Panchakarma* techniques.
3. *Shamana* (Palliative Treatment): Use of medicines and

therapies to balance *Dosha*s and prepare for surgery.

4. *Shalya* (Surgical Intervention): Precision removal or correction of pathological tissues.
5. *Ropana* (Healing): Postoperative care emphasizing wound healing and tissue regeneration.

Surgical Techniques and Instruments

Shalya Tantra describes a wide variety of techniques:

- Incision and excision: Use of scalpels, knives, and probes.
- Cauterization: Including the use of *Agnikarma* (thermal cauterization).
- Suturing: Detailed methods for wound closure using natural threads.
- *Ksharasutra* therapy: A unique Ayurvedic technique using medicated threads for fistula management.
- Fracture treatment: Reduction, immobilization, and bone setting.

The *Sushruta Samhita* catalogs over 120 surgical instruments, many of which are the precursors of modern tools.

Understanding Disease Through Doshas and Dhatus

Surgical pathology is viewed through the lens of *Dosha* imbalance and *Dhatu* (tissue) involvement. For example:

- *Vata* disorders often cause pain and impaired movement.
- *Pitta* imbalance leads to inflammation and infection.
- *Kapha* disorders cause swelling and accumulation of morbid tissues.

Healing requires not just removal of disease but restoration of *Dosha* balance and tissue nutrition.

Integration with Modern Surgery

Shalya Tantra's principles align well with modern surgical goals of:

- Minimal invasiveness
- Precision in excision
- Effective postoperative wound care
- Techniques like *Ksharasutra* therapy are now being scientifically studied for their effectiveness in treating complex anorectal fistulas, often in combination with laser procedures.

References

1. Sushruta, K. B. (2009). Sushruta Samhita, edited and translated. Chaukhamba Sanskrit Series.
2. Lad, V. (2002). Textbook of Ayurveda: Fundamental Principles. The Ayurvedic Press.
3. Singh, R. H. (2011). Ayurvedic surgical techniques: A review. Journal of Ayurveda and Integrative Medicine.
4. Gupta, A., & Kumar, A. (2018). Ksharasutra therapy in fistula-in-ano: Integrative surgical approach. Indian Journal of Surgery.

Ch. 6
Concepts of Tridosha and Dhatu in Wound Healing

In Ayurveda, the healing process is deeply rooted in the understanding of the body's fundamental biological forces—*Tridosha* (*Vata*, *Pitta*, *Kapha*) and the body's tissues or *Dhatu*s. These concepts provide a holistic framework that complements modern perspectives on tissue repair, inflammation, and regeneration.

The Tridosha: Biological Energies Governing Health

The *Tridosha* are the three primary physiological energies responsible for maintaining health and homeostasis:

- *Vata Dosha*: composed of air and ether elements; governs movement, nerve impulses, and circulation.
- *Pitta Dosha*: composed of fire and water; regulates metabolism, digestion, and inflammatory responses.
- *Kapha Dosha*: composed of earth and water; responsible for structure, lubrication, and immune defense.

Each dosha plays a crucial role in wound healing:

- *Vata* controls the transport of nutrients and removal of waste, essential for repair.
- *Pitta* regulates the inflammatory phase, heat generation, and enzymatic activity for debridement.
- *Kapha* supports tissue formation, lubrication, and granulation.

An imbalance in any *Dosha* during injury can delay healing or cause complications such as excessive inflammation or infection.

Dhatus: The Body's Building Blocks in Healing

Dhatus refer to the seven fundamental tissues that sustain life and maintain structural integrity:

1. *Rasa* (Plasma): Nourishes tissues; involved in immune response.
2. *Rakta* (Blood): Oxygenation and nutrition of tissues.
3. *Mamsa* (Muscle): Provides structure and movement.
4. *Meda* (Fat): Lubrication and cushioning.
5. *Asthi* (Bone): Structural framework and protection.
6. *Majja* (Bone marrow and nerves): Support and regeneration.
7. *Shukra* (Reproductive tissue): Vitality and regeneration.

During wound healing, these tissues undergo a sequential repair process starting from *Rasa* and *Rakta* to *Mamsa* and *Asthi*, culminating in complete tissue regeneration.

Phases of Wound Healing in Ayurvedic Context

Ayurveda conceptualizes wound healing as a coordinated effort of *Doshas* and *Dhatu*s through three main phases:

- *Shodhana* (Cleansing Phase):

Corresponds to inflammation and debridement in modern terms. *Pitta Dosha* dominates to cleanse the wound of pathogens and damaged tissues.

- *Ropana* (Healing Phase):

Kapha Dosha promotes tissue regeneration, granulation, and epithelialization. Herbal formulations aid in this phase to enhance healing.

- *Shaman* (Balancing Phase):

Vata Dosha is *Bala*nced to restore proper circulation, nerve function, and strength to the healed tissue.

Ayurvedic Interventions for Wound Healing

- Herbal Applications: Ingredients like Turmeric (Curcuma longa), *Neem* (Azadirachta indica), and Aloe vera possess anti-inflammatory, antimicrobial, and regenerative properties.
- Medicinal Oils: Oils like *Taila* are applied to nourish tissues and maintain moisture.
- *Panchakarma* Therapies: Procedures such as *Raktamokshana* (bloodletting), *Basti* (Medicated enema), *Vaman* (Emessis) and *Virechana* (purgation) help remove doshic imBalances pre and post-surgery.

Modern Science Correlation

- The inflammatory phase aligns with *Pitta*'s role in enzymatic breakdown and immune cell activation.
- Fibroblast proliferation and collagen deposition mirror *Kapha*'s constructive function.
- Nerve regeneration and restoration of tissue elasticity resonate with *Vata*'s regulation of movement and sensation.

Integrating these concepts allows surgeons to tailor interventions that not only address the mechanical aspects of healing but also support the patient's biological and energetic balance.

References

1. Sharma, H., & Clark, C. (1998). Ayurveda: The Science of Self-Healing. Lotus Press.
2. Lad, V. (2002). Textbook of Ayurveda: Fundamental Principles. The Ayurvedic Press.
3. Sumantran, V. N., & Venkatasubramanian, S. (2013). Dosha imbalances and wound healing: A review. Journal of Ayurveda and Integrative Medicine.
4. Gurtu, S., & Sharma, R. (2017). Correlating Ayurvedic wound healing with modern medicine. Indian Journal of Surgery.

Ch. 7
Agnikarma, Ksharasutra & Leech Therapy: Precision Healing Tools

Ayurveda offers a diverse array of surgical and therapeutic techniques that exemplify precision and efficacy in healing. Among these, *Agnikarma* (Thermal Cauterization), *Ksharasutra* (Medicated Thread Therapy), and Leech Therapy (*Jalaukavacharana*) stand out as specialized interventions that have withstood the test of time and continue to provide invaluable benefits, especially when integrated with modern surgical practices.

Agnikarma: The Art of Thermal Cauterization

Agnikarma is a unique Ayurvedic technique that employs controlled application of heat or cauterization to treat various diseases, especially those involving pain, inflammation, and wound management.

- Mechanism: *Agnikarma* uses heated metal instruments or herbal pastes with caustic properties to cauterize affected tissues, which promotes local healing, reduces pain, and controls bleeding.
- Applications: Effective in treating musculoskeletal pain, anal fissures, arthritis, and chronic ulcers.
- Precision: The procedure targets specific points or areas, avoiding damage to surrounding healthy tissues, thus embodying precision healing.
- Modern Correlation: *Agnikarma* can be compared to modern electrocautery or laser therapy but with a natural, less invasive approach and fewer side effects.

1. **What is Agnikarma?**

Agnikarma (fire therapy) is a para-surgical Ayurvedic procedure involving controlled thermal cauterization using heated instruments (*Shalaka*) to treat various *Vata Kapha* disorders such as musculoskeletal pain, ulcers, *fistulas*, and more.

Types of Instruments Used:

- *Tvakgata* (skin): Pippali, Ajashakriti, Cow tooth, *Shalaka* rods
- *Mamsagata* (muscle): Jambavoshtha, metals (copper, iron, gold)
- *Snayu/Asthi* (ligaments/bones): oils, ghee, wax in deeper cautery

2. **Procedure (Shalaka Method)**

- Pre-op Preparation
  - Clean and mark tender points
  - Obtain consent; confirm patient's comfort, no contraindications

- Heating the *Shalaka*
  - Heat on stove or hearth until red hot (*Shamya Dagdha Lakshana*)

- Application
  - Touch each marked point for 2–10 seconds
  - Leave ~0.5 cm between spots
  - Repeat 10–12 points to cover area without overlapping

- Signs of Correct Cauterization
  - Cracking sound, mild pain, grayish brown blisters, dry wounds

- Post Care
  - Apply aloe vera pulp, turmeric powder or cool medicated

    paste
    - Avoid wetting the area for 24 hrs

- Treatment Course
    - Each session lasts 10–30 minutes
    - 1–2 sessions for acute; 3–5 sessions over weeks for chronic issues

3. Indications
Common Indications & Disease-Specific Details

Grouped by organ-system:
A. Musculoskeletal & Pain
- Chronic low back pain (*Kateegraha*)
- Sciatica (*Gridhrasi*)

Common Indications & Disease-Specific Details
Grouped by organ-system:
Musculoskeletal & Pain
- Chronic low back pain (*Kateegraha*)
- Sciatica (*Gridhrasi*)
- Knee osteoarthritis (*Sandhigata Vāta*)
- Tennis elbow (*Kurpara Sandhigata Vāta*)
- Plantar fasciitis / calcaneal spur (*Vṛkka śūla* or *Padadāri*)
- Myofascial trigger points
- Rheumatoid nodules (though limited evidence)

B. Dermatologic / Surgery
- Corns, callosities (*Kuṣṭha – kadara*)
- Warts (*Charmakeela*)
- Keloid / hypertrophic scar (*Adhimāṃsā*)
- Small haemangioma / pyogenic granuloma

C. Vascular / Haemostasis

- Actively bleeding piles (*Arśa*)
- Varicose ulcer granulation cautery (limited)

D. ENT & Dentistry

- Recurrent aphthous ulcer (*Mukhapāka*)
- Epistaxis point cautery (*Nāsā-raktaPitta*)

E. Miscellaneous

- Non-healing sinuses (*Nāḍi-Vrana*)
- Small fibro-adenoma (experimental)

- Para-surgical uses: fistula, external piles, granulomas, early hernia

Level of Evidence: Mostly case series & small RCTs (Grade C). Not yet validated in large multicenter trials; utility is adjunctive.

3. Instruments ("Śalaka") & Heat Sources

Metal rods heated on a spirit lamp, torch or electric coil:

- Suvarna (Gold)
- Rajata (Silver)
- Tamra (Copper) – most common
- Iron, Stainless steel

Modern alternatives

- Electrocautery pencil
- CO_2 /diode laser
- Radio-frequency probe

Temperature range: 300–500 °C (copper tip glowing red). Infrared thermometer or color change used to standardize.

Tip shapes: needle-like, button-tip, spatula, flat disc – selected per lesion size & depth.

4. Step-by-Step Procedure (Standardized)

Assessment & Consent

- Rule out bleeding disorders, uncontrolled diabetes, peripheral neuropathy.
- Explain risks: burn, pain, infection, scar.

Preparation

- Shave/clean area; disinfect (povidone-iodine + spirit).
- Local/topical anaesthesia (2% lignocaine) for needles >1 mm dept

Heating

- Hold *Shalaka* with insulated forceps.
- Heat until cherry-red.
- Maintain sterile field (autoclave or single-use)

Application Techniques

- *Dāha Bindu* (dotting): multiple 2–4 mm spaced dots (for pain points).
- *Dāha Varta* (line): linear strokes along tendon (e.g., tennis elbow).
- *Dāha Valaya* (ring): circumscribe corn.
- *Dāha Pracchanna* (scraping): superficial, like dermabrasion.

Duration: < 1 sec per touch → instant blanching/brown eschar.

Post-Procedural Care

- Cool with ghee or aloe vera.
- Dress with mupirocin ointment sterile gauze for 24 h.
- NSAID ± ice next day.
- No immersion or friction for 72 h.

Follow-up

- Daily inspection first 3 d → alternate day until scab off (7–10 d).

- Reinforce physiotherapy if pain indication.

5. Therapeutic Mechanisms (Modern Explanation)

- Protein denaturation & collagen contraction → capsular tightening (seen in shoulder laxity).
- Local destruction of nociceptors → analgesia (like neurotomy).
- Counter-irritation → gate-control pain modulation.
- Micro-vascular coagulation → haemostasis, reduction of granulation tissue.
- Sterilization effect → decreases bacterial load in chronic ulcers.
- Thermal necrosis of viral-infected keratinocytes → wart resolution.

6. Evidence Snapshot (Key Studies)

Calcaneal Spur

- "Clinical evaluation of *Agnikarma* vs. steroid infiltration in heel pain" (AYU, 2015; n=60): *Agnikarma* produced ≥50% pain relief in 83% vs 70% in steroid group; better 6-month recurrence profile.

Osteoarthritis Knee

- RCT, Govt. Akola, India (J Res Ayurveda Sci 2019): *Agnikarma* + *Janu Basti* vs intra-articular hyaluronic acid. WOMAC scores improved equivalently at 8 wk; cost lower in *Agnikarma* arm. Evidence level: 2b.

Corns

- Case series of 110 lesions (Int J Ayurveda Res 2011): 96% complete resolution within one sitting; recurrence 4% at 1 yr.

Sciatica

- Small RCT (25 vs 25; JOA score) using copper rod vs pregabalin. Mixed results; *Agnikarma* group needed repeat every 3 week. Evidence inconclusive.

Limitations: Mostly single-center, small sample, lack of blinding; no head-to-head with modern RF ablation.

7. Contra-Indications & Cautions

Absolute

- Uncontrolled diabetes with neuropathy
- Peripheral vascular disease (risk of necrosis)
- Bleeding diathesis / anticoagulation
- Local cellulitis or dermal infection
- Keloid tendency if cosmetic area

Relative

- Pregnancy (avoid over abdomen/lumbar)
- Children <12 y (pain, fear)
- Immunocompromised (delayed healing)
- Over major nerves/vessels (e.g., cubital fossa)

Adverse events reported: blister, burn ulcer, post-inflammatory hypo/hyper-pigmentation, hypertrophic scar.

8. Comparison with Modern Cautery Modalities

Feature	Agnikarma (Metal Rod)	Electrocautery	RF Ablation	CO_2 Laser
Heat Source	Exogenous flame	Electric resistance	Oscillating RF current	Infrared light
Tip Temp	300–500 °C	600–1200 °C	60–90 °C (tissue)	100–200 °C
Depth Control	Manual, less precise	Good	Excellent	Excellent
Cost	Very low	Moderate	High	High
Smoke & Char	Moderate	High	Minimal	High
Electricity Need	No	Yes	Yes	Yes
Evidence	Limited	Extensive	Extensive	Extensive

Agnikarma's niche: resource-poor settings, outpatient pain procedures, cultural preference for traditional treatment.

9. Integration Into Contemporary Practice

- Can complement physiotherapy, NSAIDs, intra-articular injections.
- Must follow infection control standards (CDC blood-borne pathogen protocol).
- Always document lesion size, depth, temperature used, number of dots, adverse effects.

Medicolegal note (India): Ministry of AYUSH recognizes *Agnikarma* under *Shalya Tantra*. Practitioners require BAMS with training. Outside India, local regulations vary; performing without license may be illegal.

10. Practical Tips (Clinical Pearls)

1. Use infrared thermometer (non-contact) to standardize tip at 450 °C for musculoskeletal lesions; prevents over-burning.

2. For heel spur, apply 4–6 dots along medial fascial band, not over calcaneal fat pad (risk of ulcer).
3. In corns, perform ring diathermy (*dāha valaya*) and core excision same sitting.
4. Always keep cold sterile saline nearby; if depth exceeds dermis, immediate cooling prevents tissue necrosis.
5. Offer tetanus prophylaxis if status uncertain.

11. Suggested Learning Resources & Visuals

- Illustrated Atlas of *Agnikarma Shalaka*s – Gujarat Ayurved University, 2020.
- Video demonstrations (YouTube channels: CCRAS, "AyuSoft Learning") – look for "*Agnikarma* on Tennis Elbow".
- Textbook: "*Shalya Tantra* – The Surgical Art of Ayurveda" by A. M. Athavale, 2018; Chapter 18.

Key Takeaways

- *Agnikarma* is a low-technology form of thermal cauterization used primarily for pain, dermatologic lesions, and haemostasis.
- Clinical evidence is growing but remains limited; best applied as adjunct to guideline-based modern care.
- Proper case selection, asepsis, temperature control, and post-procedure care are critical to minimize complications.

This tool is designed to support clinical reasoning. Always apply individual judgment, patient context, and institutional protocols when making decisions.

4. Mechanism of Action

- Enhances local circulation, stimulates tissue metabolism
- Opens micro-channels (*Srotas*) to clear blockages
- Analgesic effect via nociceptive modulation
- Induces coagulative necrosis and controlled healing

6. Clinical Examples & Case Reports

A. Corn (Clavi) Treatment

Case Study: 45 year old female with plantar corn

Method: Heated *Shalaka* in circular motion

Outcome: Relief within 1 week; full resolution in 8 weeks; no recurrence

B. Plantar Fasciitis (Vata Kantaka)

Randomized Study: *Agnikarma* vs *Siravedha* (veinletting) in 40 patients

Results: 90.5% relief in *Agnikarma* vs 88.3% in *Siravedha*

C. Sciatica Pain

"*Agnikarma* offers substantial pain relief... The application of heat helps in releasing endorphins... providing immediate comfort."

7. Integrative Approach

Combine with herbal sitz baths, medicated oils (e.g., Murivenna)

Use alongside internal treatments for chronic cases or ulcer healing

Follow Ayurveda's *Dosha Prakriti* principles for patient selection

8. Key Advantages

- Minimally invasive, non surgical
- Rapid pain relief, minimal bleeding
- Economical, performed on OPD basis
- Low risk of recurrence when correctly administered

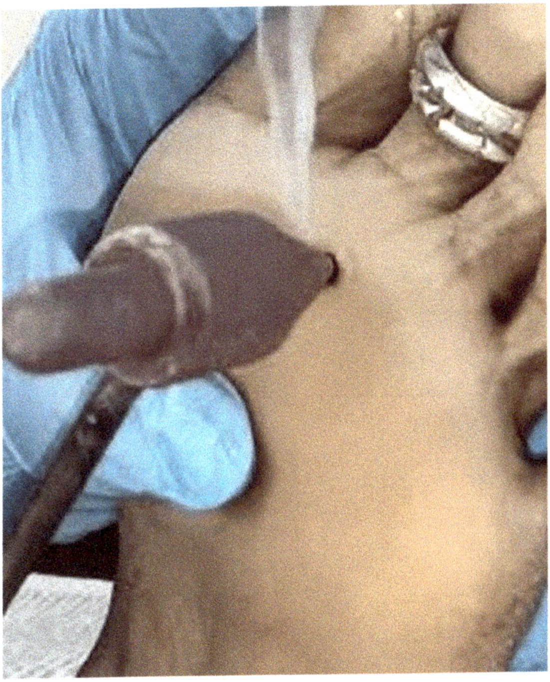

Agni-karma for corn

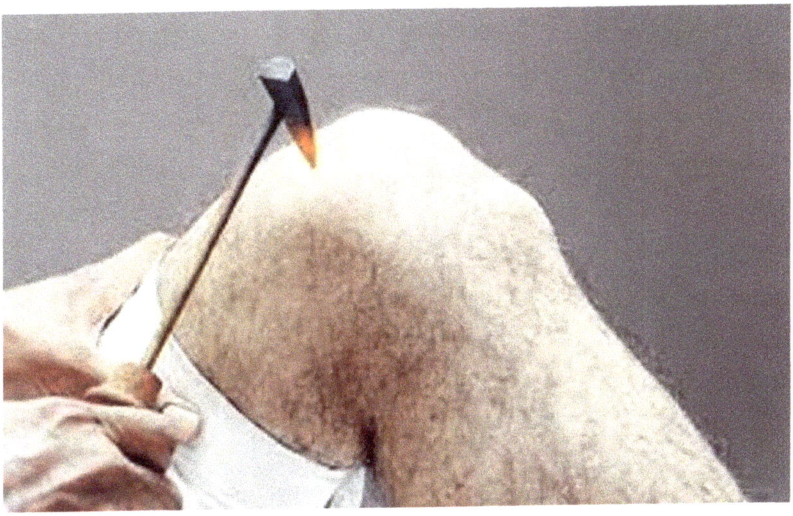

Agnikarma for knee pain

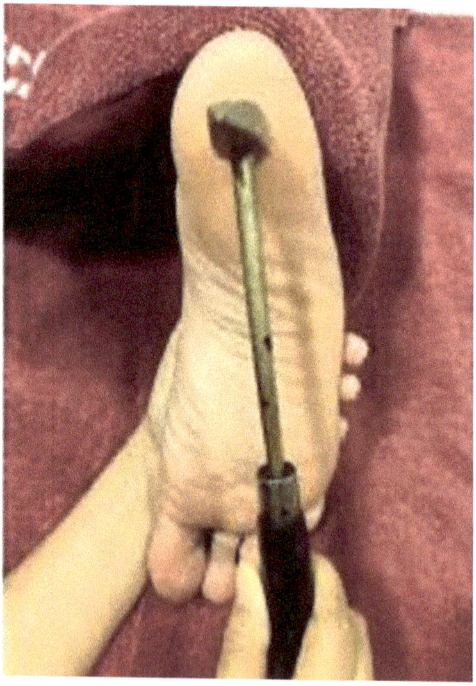

Agnikarma for calcaneal spur

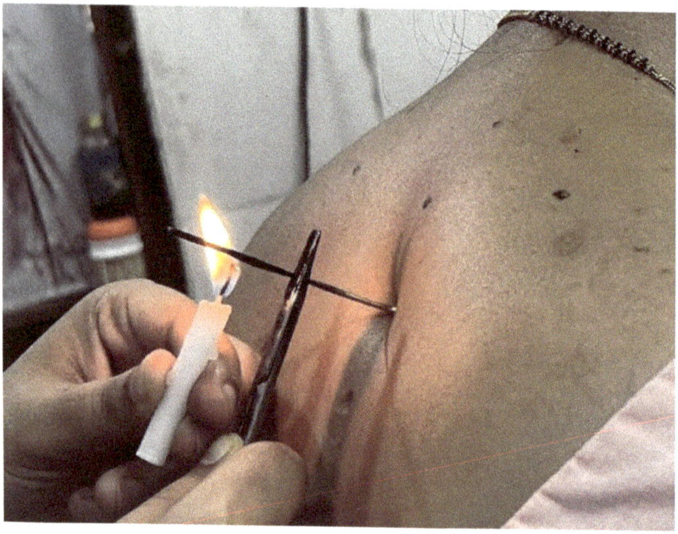

Agnikarma for cervical radiculopathy

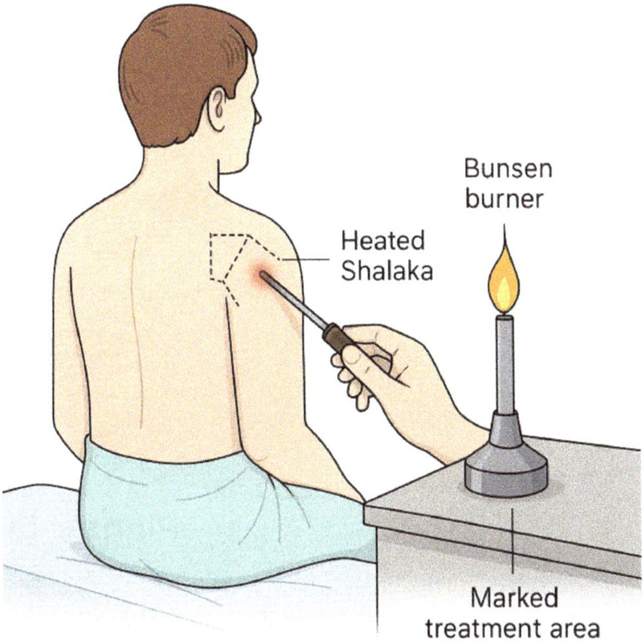

Close-up of *Shalaka* tip and skin interaction

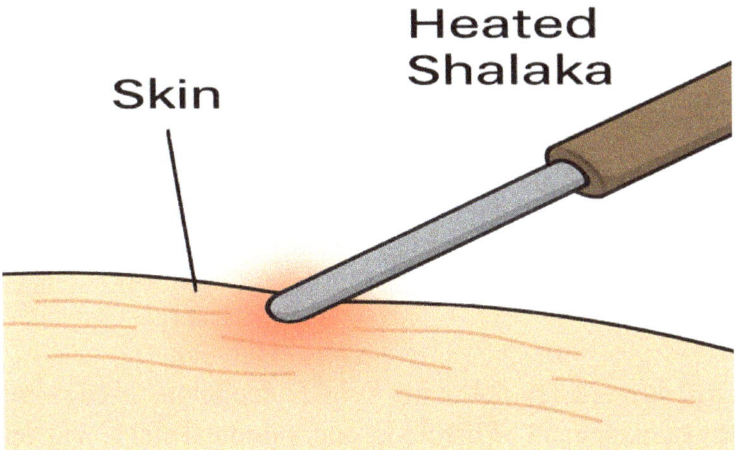

Sequence: marking → heating → application → post-care
Visuals for corn and plantar fascia treatment

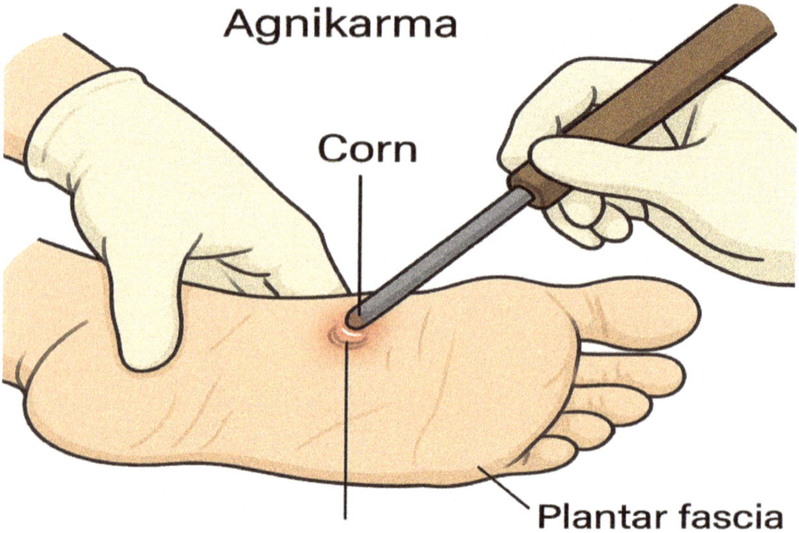

Case timeline sheets (pre- and post-treatment)

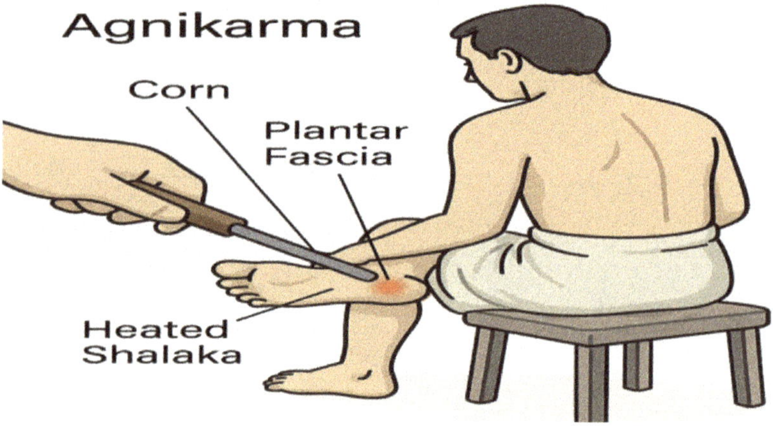

Ksharasutra is a revolutionary surgical technique used primarily for the management of fistula-in-ano, pilonidal sinus, and certain types of abscesses.

Ksharasutra Therapy: *Ksharasutra*: Medicated Thread Therapy

An Advanced Ayurvedic Technique

1. Introduction

Ksharasutra is a para-surgical Ayurvedic technique used primarily for the treatment of anorectal disorders such as fistula-in-ano (*Bhagandara*), piles (*Arsha*), and sinuses (*Nadi Vrana*). It involves the application of a specially prepared medicated thread to excise and heal the diseased tract with minimal tissue damage and recurrence.

2. Historical References

Described in classical texts like *Sushruta Samhita* and *Charaka Samhita* under the term "*Kshara Karma*".

Sushruta recommended this for non-healing sinuses and fistulas.

3. Composition of Ksharasutra

A *Ksharasutra* is a surgical linen thread (Barbour Linen No. 20) coated with multiple layers of specific Ayurvedic drugs:

- ***Composition:*** The thread is coated with Ayurvedic alkaline substances (*Kshara*) derived from plants like Achyranthes aspera and Snuhi latex, possessing caustic, antimicrobial, and healing properties.
- ***Procedure:*** The medicated thread is passed through the fistulous tract, where it gradually cuts through the tissue while simultaneously promoting healing and preventing infection.
- ***Advantages:*** Minimally invasive, low recurrence rate, reduced postoperative pain, and no need for complex surgery.
- ***Scientific Validation:*** Numerous clinical studies confirm the safety and efficacy of *Ksharasutra* therapy, making it a valuable tool in integrative proctology.

Coating Layer	Material Used	Purpose
1st–7th	Guggulu solution	Binding base
8th–14th	Apamarga Kshara (Achyranthes aspera)	Cauterization and debridement
15th–21st	Haridra (Curcuma longa) powder	Antiseptic and wound healing

Advanced Modifications:

Use of *Katuki* (Picrorhiza kurroa), *Neem*, or *Triphala*-infused variants for specific infections.

Chromic catgut *Ksharasutra* for faster absorption in internal tracts.

4. Mechanism of Action

Cauterization (*Ksharana*): Chemical cautery of unhealthy tissue.

Dissection: Gradual cutting of the tract.

Healing: Promotes healthy granulation and fibrosis to prevent recurrence.

5. Indications

Condition	Description
Fistula-in-ano	Primary and secondary tracts
Piles (*Arsha*)	Internal and external hemorrhoids
Pilonidal sinus	Recurrent infected sinuses in sacrococcygeal area
Anal polyps	Pedunculated lesions
Non-healing wounds	Sinuses and cavities

6. Contraindications

Acute abscess with active pus.

Patients with bleeding disorders, diabetes mellitus (uncontrolled).

Malignant or tubercular tracts.

7. Procedure

a. Preoperative:

Anorectal examination

Fistulogram or MRI in complex *fistulas*

Shodhana & *Deepana* (internal cleansing) with *Triphala* or Panchatikta decoction

b. Operative:

Anesthesia: Local, spinal, or saddle block

Probing of the tract

Thread placement through entire tract

Tightening or replacement every 7 days

c. Postoperative:

Sitz bath with *Triphala Kwatha*

Jatyadi Taila / *Panchavalkala* ointment

Analgesics and wound care

8. Rate of Cutting

Average cutting rate: 0.5–1 cm/week

Depends on the tightness of the thread and tract complexity

9. Advantages

Minimally invasive

Low recurrence rate (~3–7%)

Cost-effective

Day-care procedure

10. Complications

Complication	Prevention/Management
Thread breakage	Avoid excess tightening
Infection	Aseptic dressing; antibiotic cover if needed
Incontinence	Avoid sphincter damage via imaging-guided placement
Pain or spasm	Sitz bath + local analgesic oil

11. Clinical Evidence

ICMR Trials: Showed 96% cure rate in simple fistulae.

AIIMS Studies: Reported significantly fewer recurrences compared to Fistulectomy.

12. Integration with Modern Proctology

Used alongside MRI-guided diagnosis, laser ablation, and endoscopic visualization in complex cases.

Ksharasutra-ligation with diode laser hybrid technique emerging.

13. Case Vignette Example

Case: 35-year-old male with low transsphincteric fistula

MRI: Single tract, 3.5 cm

Treatment: *Ksharasutra* insertion under spinal anesthesia

Follow-up: Weekly tightening x 4 weeks

Outcome: Complete healing, no recurrence after 18 months

14. High-Resolution Medical Illustration

Anal fistula represents a chronic, granulation-lined tract between the anorectal canal and perianal skin, almost always arising from an infected anal crypt–gland unit. Definitive therapy must eradicate sepsis, close the internal opening, and preserve continence.

Over the last decade several sphincter-sparing procedures (LIFT, VAAFT, FiLaC, OTSC, stem cells) have emerged. In many parts of South-Asia, an Ayurvedic variant—IFTAK (Interception of Fistulous Tract with Application of *Kṣārasūtra*)—is in use as a modification of the classical *Kṣārasūtra* therapy to shorten healing time and reduce post-operative pain while maintaining low recurrence.

IFTAK: Concept & Rationale

1. Interception: The tract is "short-circuited" by laying open only a 1–2 cm segment at the level of the internal opening and intersphincteric plane, thereby disconnecting the proximal septic focus from the external cutaneous opening.
2. *Kṣārasūtra* Placement: A medicated thread (coated in Snuhi latex, *Apāmārga* and *Haridrā* powders, later dipped in alkaline ash) is passed only through the intercepted short segment instead of the entire tract. The thread's caustic, antimicrobial, and mild cutting action promotes fibrous healing while minimising division of external sphincter muscle.

Mechanistically, IFTAK parallels the surgical principle of LIFT (ligation/interception in the inter-sphincteric plane), but uses a chemically active seton rather than suture ligation.

Indications & Patient Selection

Appropriate for:

- Primary or recurrent low to mid-level trans- or inter-sphincteric fistulae (Parks types II–III)
- Tracts without high supralevator extension or multiple secondary branches > 3 cm from midline
- Patients motivated for weekly outpatient thread changes

Contra-indications:

- High supra-sphincteric, extra-sphincteric, or horseshoe fistula

- Active Crohn's disease, tuberculosis, malignancy
- Incontinence baseline, poor wound healing (uncontrolled diabetes)
- Pregnancy, bleeding diathesis

Pre-operative Work-up

1. Proctoscopy & methylene blue test to confirm internal opening.
2. MRI pelvis or 3-D endoanal ultrasound for complex or recurrent tracts.
3. Baseline labs (CBC, glucose, HIV/HBV/HCV).
4. Bowel prep: enema (Ayurvedic *Triphalā Kwātha* or standard PEG).
5. Consent emphasising need for repeated thread changes and rare risk of incontinence (< 1–3 %).

Step-by-Step Technique (Operative Field: Lithotomy, Spinal ± IV sedation)

Step	**Key Points**
1. Identification	Probe tract; inject 1–2 ml hydrogen peroxide/ methylene blue through external opening; locate internal opening at dentate line.
2. Small curvilinear incision	0.5–1 cm incision at 4 or 8 o'clock just lateral to anal verge over inter-sphincteric plane.
3. Interception & derailment	Dissect to expose tract; divide it between two haemostats, leaving proximal limb attached to internal opening.
4. Curettage	Gently scrape granulation tissue within tract segments.

5. Kṣārasūtra threading	Feed the medicated thread through internal opening ->intercepted tract -> out via the new skin incision, not the external cutaneous opening. Secure with loose knot.
6. External limb dealt with	Often excised/curetted and left open for drainage.
7. Dressing	Betadine gauze / Jatyādi tailam soaked pack. No anal packing.

Average operative time: 15–25 min. Blood loss negligible.

Post-operative Protocol

1. Sitz bath (lukewarm water + *Panchavalkala* decoction) × 15 min TID.
2. Oral analgesia: NSAID ± Ayurvedic *Gandhak Rasayana.*
3. Broad-spectrum antibiotic x 3–5 days (co-amoxyclav or ciprofloxacin + metronidazole).
4. Stool softener: Polyethylene glycol or *Triphalā Churna.*
5. Weekly OPD thread change: Replace *Kṣārasūtra* until it "cheese-wires" and drops off (2–3 weeks average).
6. Observe for bleeding, cellulitis, fever.

Return to normal activity generally within 2–3 days.

Healing, Follow-up & Outcomes

- Time to complete healing: 4–6 weeks (vs 10–12 weeks in conventional *Kṣārasūtra*).
- Reported recurrence: 2–8 % at 1-year in small prospective cohorts (n = 40–120).
- Continence scores (Wexner): Essentially unchanged in > 95 %.
- Pain scores (VAS): Significantly lower after first 48 h versus classical method (Patil et al., AYU 2022).
- Work days lost: Median 5 vs 12 days.

Level of evidence is limited (uncontrolled series; no RCTs). Nonetheless, early data compare favourably with LIFT (recurrence ~ 6–17 %) and VAAFT (recurrence ~ 20 %).

Complications & Red Flags

Complication	Prevention / Management
Premature thread drop	Ensure adequate weekly replacement; if gap forms, place fresh thread immediately.
Secondary abscess	Early recognition; incision & drainage ± culture based antibiotics.
Bleeding	Usually minor; persistent bleeding warrants cauterisation.
Incontinence (rare)	Proper plane dissection; avoid external sphincter division.
Recurrence	Re-evaluate with MRI; consider LIFT, FiLaC, advancement flap.

Urgent attention for: sudden purulent discharge with systemic signs, new continence issues, uncontrolled pain.

Comparison with Other Sphincter-Sparing Procedures

Parameter	IFTAK	LIFT	VAAFT	FiLaC
Anaesthesia	Spinal / LA	RA / GA	GA	GA/RA
Equipment cost	Low	Low	High (scope)	Moderate (laser)
Healing time	4–6 wk	4–8 wk	6–10 wk	4–6 wk
Continence risk	< 3 %	< 5 %	< 2 %	< 2 %
Recurrence (meta-mean)	6 %	10 %	20 %	13 %
Out-patient thread change	Yes	No	No	No

Patient Education Pearls

"In simple terms, we will cut and clean just a small segment of the track inside, place a medicated thread that slowly removes diseased tissue and promotes healthy healing. You will come weekly for thread change; most patients heal in about a month, can walk from day one, and rarely lose bowel control. Keep stools soft, do warm baths, and report fever, swelling, or loss of control immediately."

Evidence & Guideline Snapshot

- Shukla et al., J-Research Ayur Sci 2018 – Prospective n = 54; healing 5.3 ± 1.1 wk; recurrence 3.7 %.
- Patil et al., AYU 2022 – Randomised 72 pts (IFTAK vs classical); pain & healing significantly better in IFTAK ($p < 0.05$).
- No inclusion yet in European Society of Coloproctology (ESCP) 2023 guidelines; regarded as "emerging regional technique with limited but promising data."

More high-quality RCTs and long-term (> 3 yr) follow-up are needed before broad adoption in western guidelines.

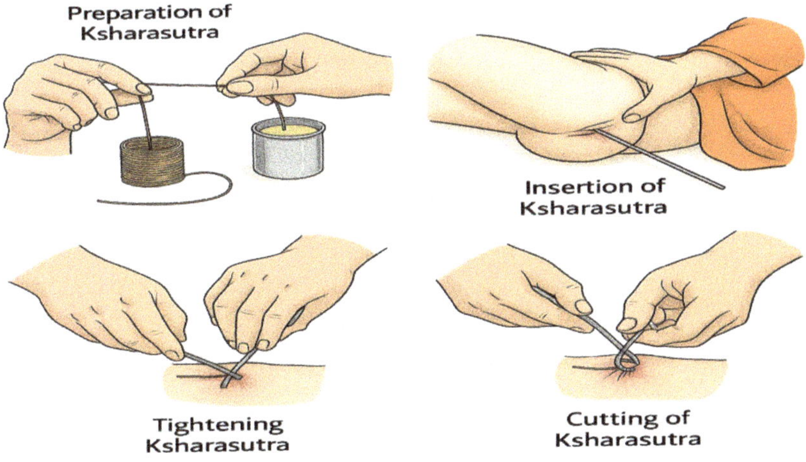

KSHARASUTRA

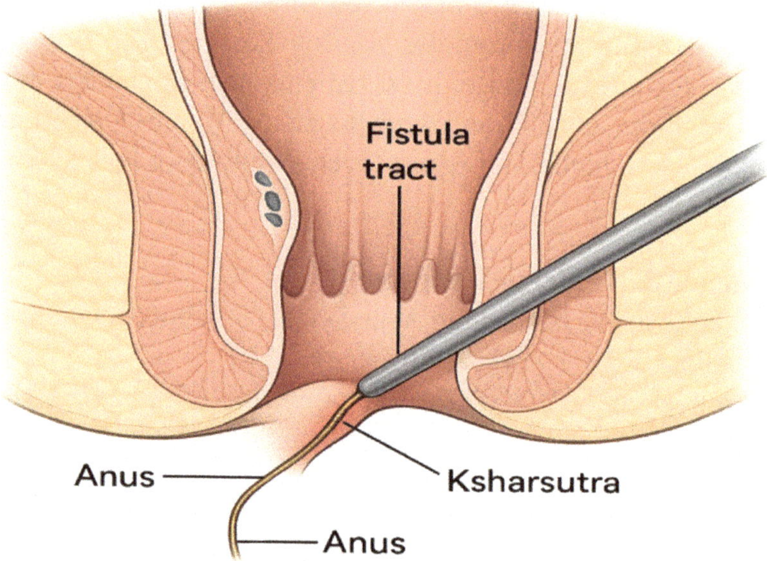

Ksharasutra Treatment for Fistulain in Anus

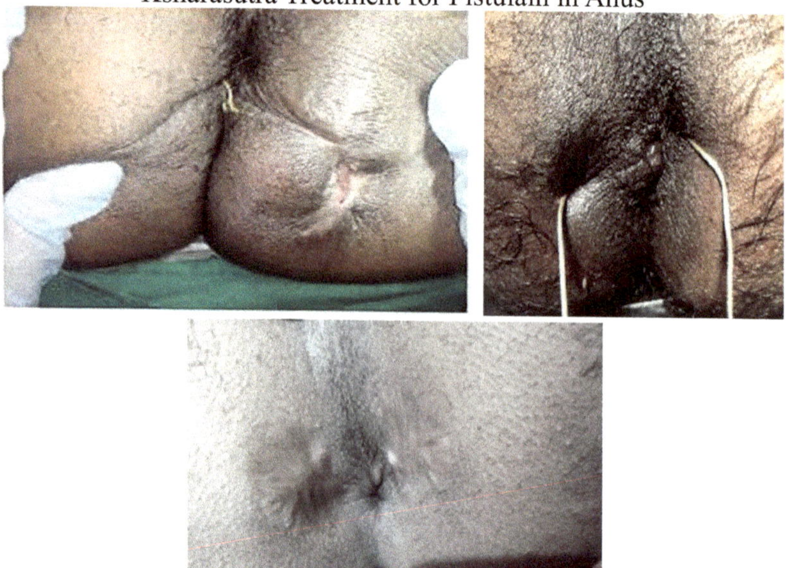

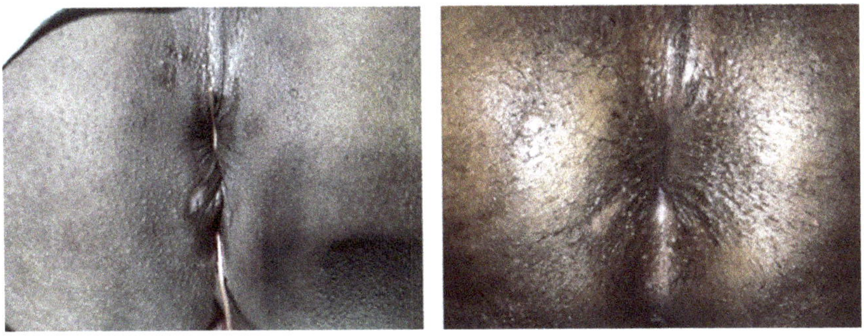

Post Iftak

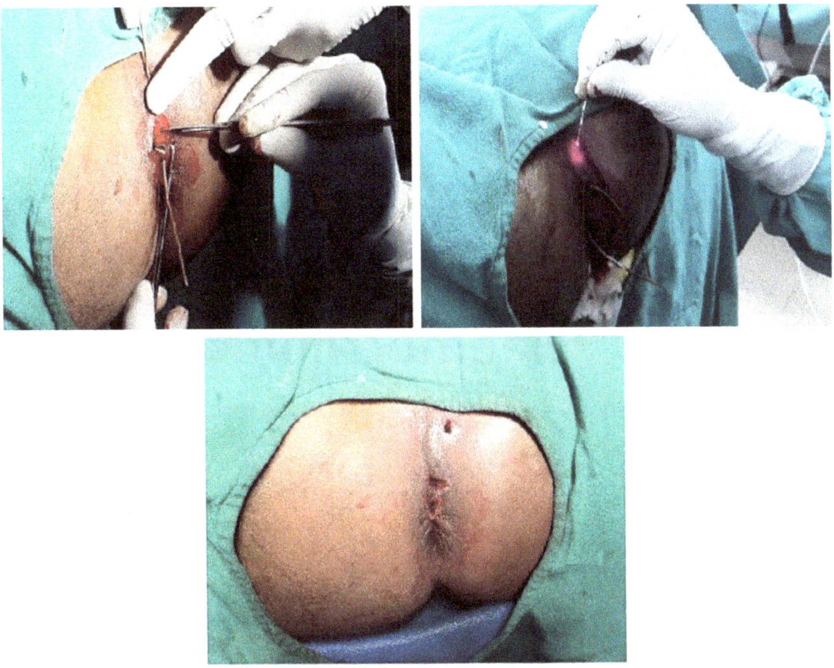

Laser Ablation of Fistulain in Ano With Ksharasutra

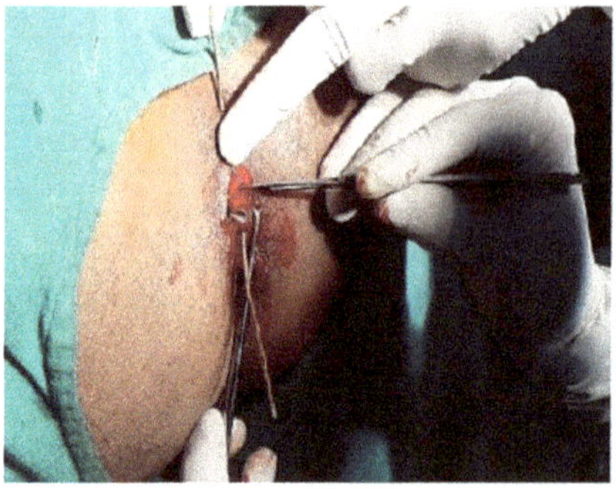
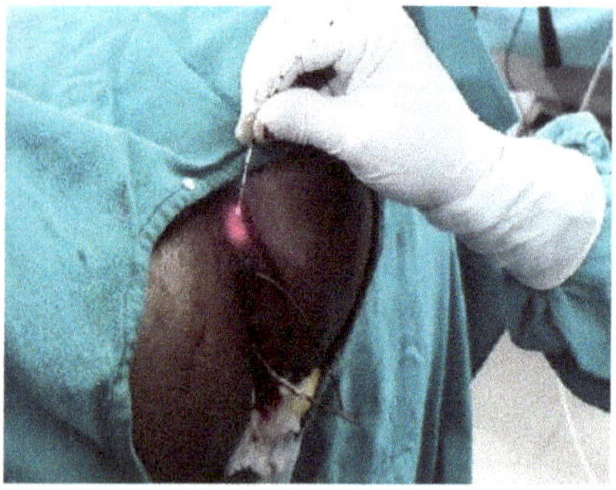
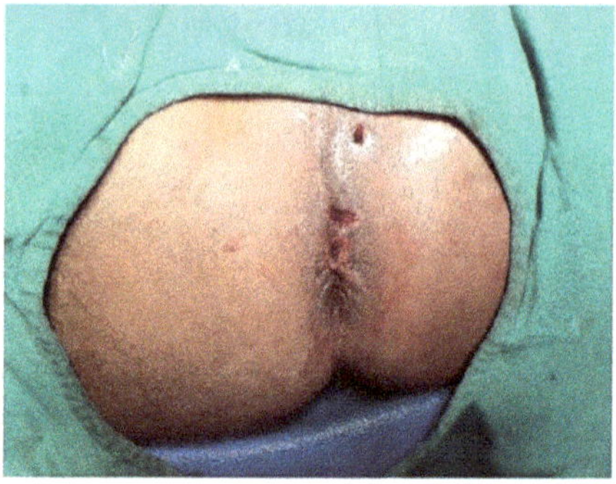

Haemorrhoids

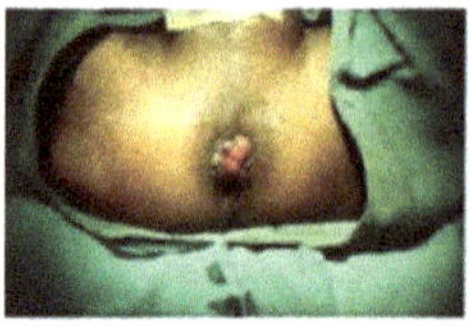

Haemorrhoids

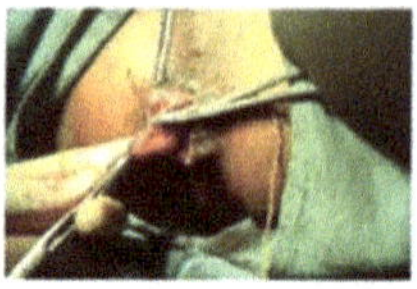
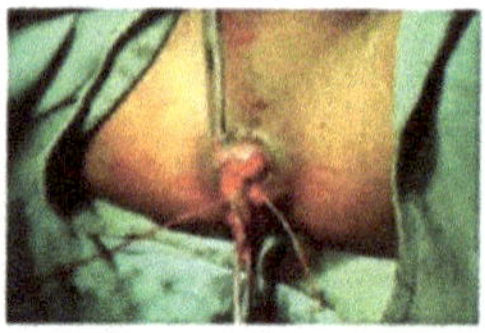

Ligation of haemorrhoid with kshara sutra

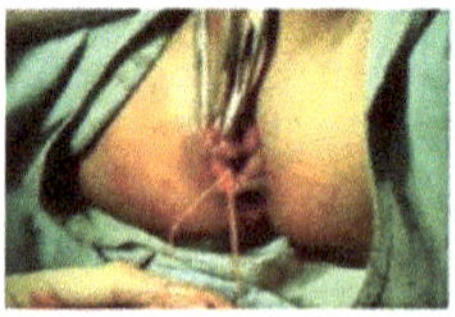

Tying of knot

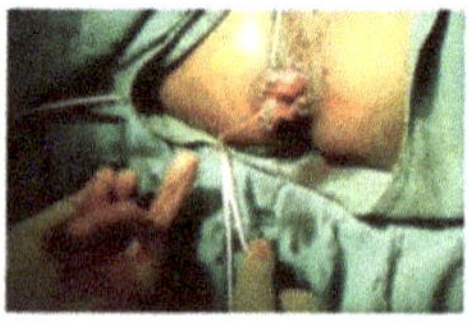

Cutting of thread

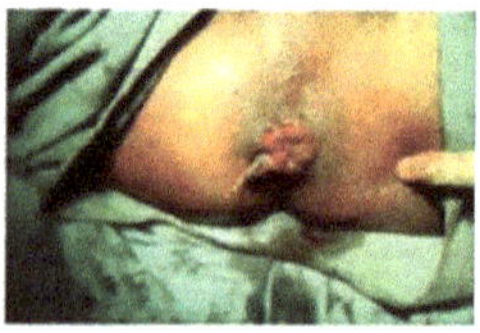

Ligated haemorrhoid

Leech Therapy (Jalaukavacharana): Nature's Healing Touch
Leech Therapy (Jalaukavacharana)
Integration of Ayurveda and Modern Science for Bloodletting and Detoxification

1. Introduction

Leech therapy (*Jalaukavacharana*) is a biological bloodletting procedure used in Ayurveda, classified under *Raktamokshana* – a *Panchakarma* modality. It is especially useful in *Pitta* and Rakta-vitiated conditions.

Classical Source:

स्निग्धोष्णे सति दूष्ये स्याद्रक्तदुष्टि ज्वरादिषु।
शस्तं रक्तं विमोक्तव्यमिति सिद्धान्त निर्मितिः।।

(*Charaka Samhita*, Sutra*Sthana* 24/18)

"In *Pitta*-predominant diseases, vitiated blood should be removed to alleviate symptoms."

2. Types of Leeches (Jalauka Bheda)

Type	Description	Nature	Usage
Savisha	Wild, venomous	Irritative	Not used
Nirvisha	Non-venomous (medicinal)	Safe, therapeutic	Used in therapy

Medicinal leeches (Hirudo medicinalis) are commonly used in clinical settings today.

3. Properties of Leech Saliva

Leech saliva contains >100 bioactive substances:

Component	Action
Hirudin	Potent anticoagulant
Bdellins	Anti-inflammatory
Eglins	Protease inhibitors
Hyaluronidase	Enhances tissue permeability
Calin	Platelet aggregation inhibitor
Destabilase	Dissolves blood clots

These help reduce inflammation, pain, vascular congestion, and improve microcirculation.

4. Indications

Ayurvedic Condition	Modern Equivalent
Vatarakta	Gout, vasculitis
Dushta Vrana	Non-healing wounds
Pittaja Netra Roga	Eye diseases with inflammation
Granthi	Cysts, nodules
Arsha	Hemorrhoids (esp. thrombosed piles)
Vidradhi	Abscess
Kotha / Dushta Vrana	Gangrene, ischemic ulcers

Reference:

"*Jalauka Nirharati Doshitam Raktam, Snehavat Krishyam Yatha Tailam*" (*Sushruta Samhita, Sutra Sthana* 13/4)

"Leeches draw out vitiated blood, just as oil is pulled out by absorbent material."

5. Contraindications

- Anemia (*Pandu*)
- Severe bleeding disorders (*RaktaPitta*)
- Cachexia, immunosuppressed states
- Pregnancy, children under 5
- Snake/Scorpion bite (*Savisha* conditions)

6. Procedure (Jalauka Avacharana Vidhi)

A. Pre-Procedural Care

- Select healthy leeches (4–6 cm, active, blackish)
- Clean leeches in turmeric water (antimicrobial)
- Prepare the site (shave, wash with lukewarm water)

B. Main Procedure

Step	Action
Application	Place leech on affected site (painful or inflamed area)
Sucking begins	Leech attaches, sucks blood for 20–45 mins
Detachment	Once full, leech detaches naturally or with turmeric
Post-care	Site cleaned with antiseptic + Jatyadi taila application
Leech care	Induce vomiting by turmeric solution; store in fresh water

Evidence & Indications (Modern + Ayurveda Alignment)

Category	Classical Indications	Contemporary Evidence / Use
Vascular / Congestive	*Vardhana* (local swelling), *śonita dushti*	Post-replant venous congestion (Grade A evidence; 2016 Cochrane)
Musculoskeletal / Pain	*Sandhigata vata, gridhrasi*	Knee OA pain ↓ (RCTs: Michalsen 2008, Bäcker 2022)
Dermatologic / Ulcers	*Vidradhi, dushta vraṇa* (chronic ulcers)	Mixed evidence; small pilot trials for diabetic foot ulcers
ENT / Ophthalmology	*Netra-roga, karṇa-śūla*	Case reports only
Miscellaneous	Hypertension, headache (*rakta-gata pitta)*	Insufficient evidence

Strength of Recommendation:

- Strong (venous congestion)
- Weak to Very Low (others)

Contra-indications & Red-Flag Precautions

Absolute

- Hemophilia or inherited coagulopathy
- Severe anemia (Hb < 8 g/dL)
- Uncontrolled DM with sepsis risk
- Immunocompromised / neutropenia
- Active anticoagulation (INR > 3.0)

Relative

- Pregnancy, children < 10 y, severe hypotension
- Allergy to leech saliva proteins (rare but reportable)

Red Flags During Therapy

- Excessive bleeding > 2 hrs
- Cellulitis or rapidly spreading erythema (Aeromonas hydrophila infection)
- Signs of anaphylaxis

Prophylaxis: oral ciprofloxacin or TMP-SMX targeting Aeromonas (IDSA 2023).

Procedure at a Glance (Hybrid Protocol)

1. Patient consent and Hb/platelet baseline.
2. Select "non-toxic" leeches (*Suśruta: śānta-tīkṣṇāḥ*). In practice: Hirudo medicinalis from certified bio-farms.
3. Local cleansing with chlorhexidine; avoid alcohol (repellent).
4. Gentle scarification or sugar drop to initiate attachment.
5. Average feed ~ 20 mL; detach when satiated or after 30 min using sterile saline.
6. Post-site compression 10 min; sterile dressing with pressure.
7. Observe at 15-min intervals first hour; vital signs, bleeding.
8. Dispose single-use leeches as biohazard (regulatory *Mandate*).
9. Prophylactic antibiotic course 3–5 days.
10. Re-apply per indication (e.g., congested flap every 6–8 h, max 2–3 days).

- Hb, hematocrit daily if multiple leeches
- Wound cultures if discharge
- HbA1c in diabetics; nutrition optimization
- Document pain scores (VAS), functional outcome (KOOS for knee OA)

7. **Duration & Frequency**

- 1–2 sittings/week depending on condition
- Total: 3–8 sessions for chronic condition
- Healing visible within 3–4 sitting

8. Advantages

- Natural, biological debridement
- Promotes oxygenation, healing
- Safe in vascular disorders
- Useful when surgery is contraindicated
- Non-invasive, minimal pain

9. Complications & Management

Complication	Cause	Management
Excess bleeding	Over-attachment	Cold compression, alum paste
Allergy	Protein in saliva	Antihistamines, stop therapy
Infection	Improper hygiene	Antibiotics, antiseptic care

10. Case Vignette Example

- Patient: Male, 58 yrs – Thrombosed external hemorrhoid
- Symptoms: Acute pain, swelling, bluish discoloration
- Treatment: Leech application on perianal site × 3 sessions
- Outcome: Pain relief in 24 hrs; swelling reduced by 80% in 72 hrs

11. Integration with Laser Proctology

Leech therapy is complementary to:

- Laser hemorrhoidoplasty: Use leech for post-op pain or in thrombosed piles
- Perianal abscess drainage: Use leeches in low immunity where surgery is risky
- Wound bed preparation: Leech in ischemic areas before skin grafting.

12. High-Resolution Illustrations

I can generate custom images for:

- Leech attachment to skin (macro view)
- Anorectal leech therapy site
- Leech anatomy with salivary gland labelin
- Leech detachment and post-care process

Leech therapy involves the controlled application of medicinal leeches to affected areas to remove impure blood and promote healing.

- Historical Use: Documented extensively in Ayurvedic texts for detoxification and treatment of blood disorders.
- Mechanism: Leeches secrete a complex mixture of bioactive substances including anticoagulants (hirudin), vasodilators, and anesthetics which improve blood circulation and reduce inflammation.
- Modern Applications: Used in reconstructive surgery, treatment of varicose veins, chronic wounds, and certain skin diseases.
    - Integrative Benefits: Leech therapy supports microcirculation and tissue regeneration, complementing surgical healing especially in complicated wounds and flap surgeries.

Integrative Application in Surgical Practice

- Combining *Agnikarma* with Laser Therapy: Using controlled heat to enhance laser precision in tissue ablation and pain management.
- *Ksharasutra* alongside Minimal Invasive Surgery: Employing medicated threads to treat *fistulas* while minimizing surgical trauma.
- Leech Therapy in Postoperative Care: Applying leeches to improve venous circulation and reduce postoperative edema and infection.

Leech Therapy for Skin Diseases

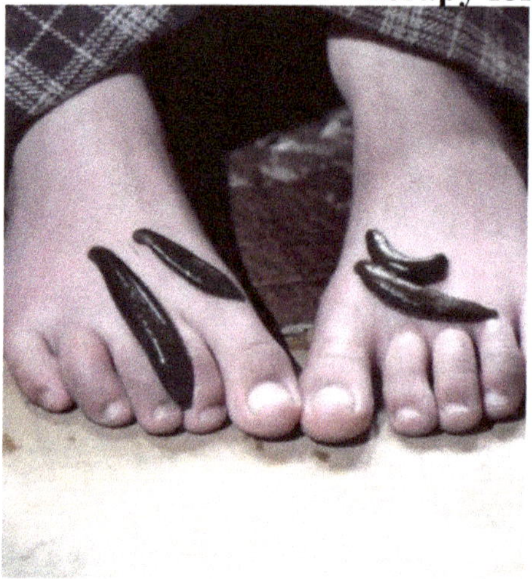

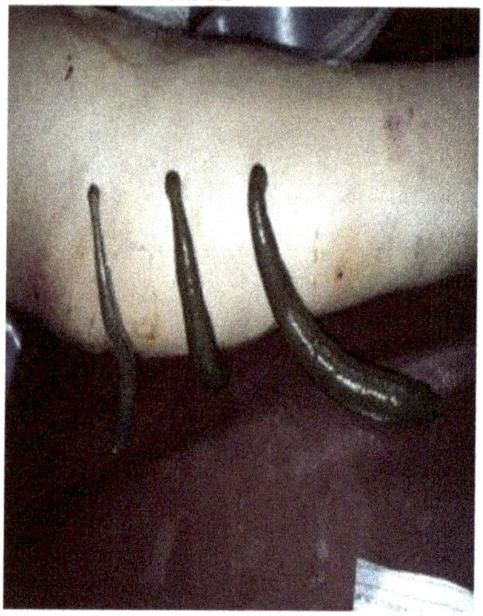

Leech Therapy for Non Healing Wound

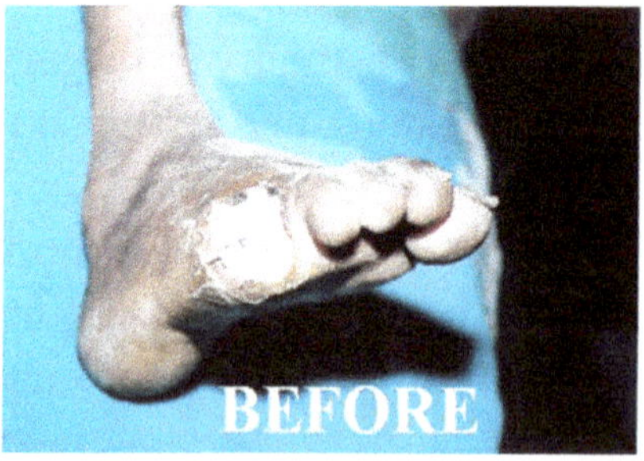

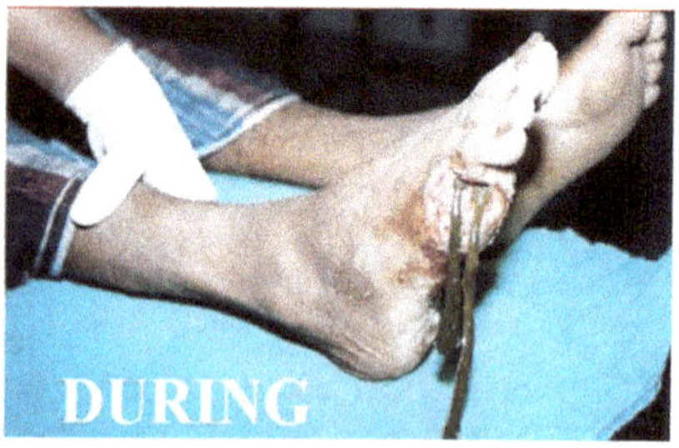

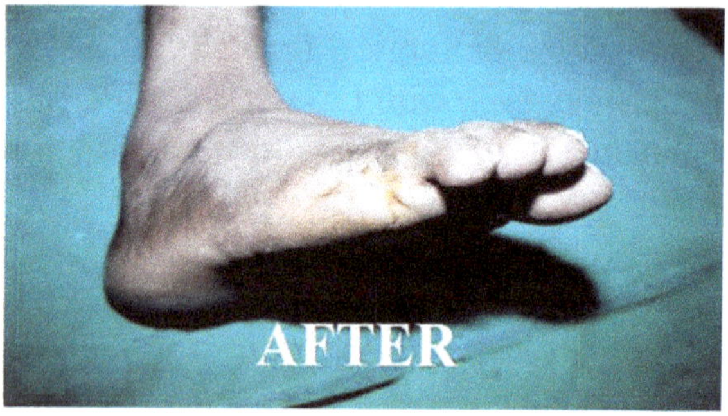

Leech Therapy for Eczema

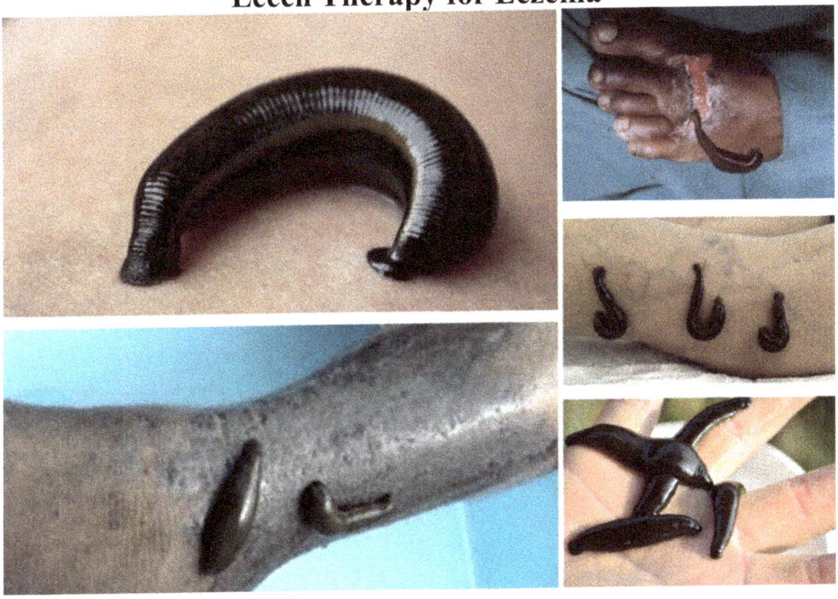

Leech Therapy for Thrombosed Piles

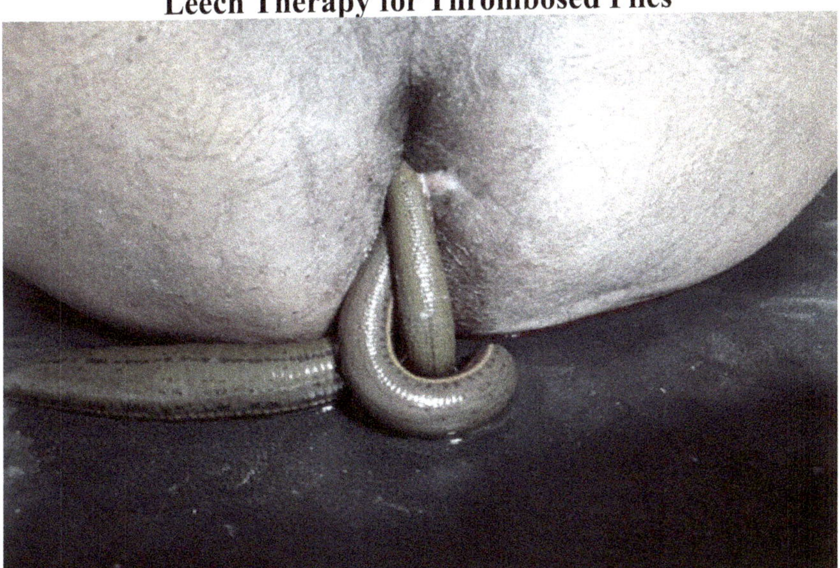

Where Does Leech Therapy (Jalaukāvacaraṇa) Fit?

Rationale

- Ayurvedic premise: local venous congestion → "vitiated rakta" that can be removed by blood-letting.
- Modern hypothesis: transient local decongestion + antithrombotic/anti-inflammatory salivary peptides (hirudin, calin, bdellins) may reduce pain and oedema.

Technique (Ayurvedic texts)

- Species: Hirudo medicinalis or Indian species (*Hirudinaria granulosa*) 2-4 leeches applied per session.
- Placement: perianal skin adjacent to the haemorrhoidal plexus, left until satiation (20-40 min), then detached with saline/turmeric paste.
- Sessions: usually weekly × 3–4.
- Concomitant oral *Triphala Guggulu* or topical *Jatyadi Taila* often prescribed.

Current Evidence (2020–2024)

Study	Design	N	Comparator	Outcome	Limitations
Saxena et al, AYU 2021	RCT	60	RBL	Similar symptomatic relief at 4 wks; more rapid pain reduction with leech; higher recurrence at 6 mo	Single-centre, unblinded
Sharma et al, J Ethnopharm 2022	Pilot RCT	40	Sitz bath + flavonoids	Greater reduction in pain/pruritus day 3; no diff. at 1 mo	Under-powered
Bhardwaj et al, Complement Ther Clin Pract 2023	Prospective cohort	75	None	70 % complete symptom control at 2 wk in grade II piles	No control, subjective endpoints

- No trials with grade III–IV prolapse.
- No guideline (ASCRS 2022, NICE CKS 2023) recommends

leeching; evidence rated very low (GRADE ↓↓).

Safety & Contra-indications

- Infective: Aeromonas hydrophila sepsis (prophylax with 3rd-gen ceph +/- fluoroquinolone in immunocompromised).
- Bleeding: average 10–20 mL per leech; avoid in anemia (Hb < 10 g/dL), coagulopathy, anticoagulation/antiplatelet therapy.
- Allergic reactions, anaphylaxis (rare).
- Transmission of blood-borne pathogens if leeches reused—strict single-use & medical-grade sourcing *Manda*tory.
- Pregnancy: no data; generally avoided.

Practical Algorithm (If Considering Integrative Use)

1. Confirm grade I–II haemorrhoids, rule out fissure, fistula, IBD, malignancy.
2. Optimise conservative measures first (≥ 4 wks fibre 25–30 g/d + 2 L water, topical steroids ≤ 7 days, flavonoids).
3. Shared decision-making: discuss standard office procedures vs. leech therapy; explain limited evidence & off-guideline status.
4. Pre-procedure checks: CBC, PT/INR, HIV/HBsAg/HCV, consent for non-standard therapy.
5. Leech session in minor OT with sterile drapes, prophylactic 500 mg ciprofloxacin PO 1 h pre-procedure (expert opinion).
6. Post-session pressure dressing × 6 h; monitor vitals; discharge same day with analgesia (paracetamol/NSAID).
7. Review at 1 wk, 4 wk. Escalate to RBL or surgical intervention for persistent bleeding, prolapse, or thrombosis.

Red Flags / When Not to Delay Conventional Care

- Acute profuse rectal bleeding (Hb drop > 2 g/dL)
- Strangulated, thrombosed external piles with severe pain > 72 h
- Suspicion of colorectal carcinoma (weight loss, iron

deficiency, mass)

- Immunocompromised host or pregnancy

References

1. Singh, R.H., & Rastogi, S. (2010). Agnikarma: An Ayurvedic technique of thermal cauterization. Ayurveda Journal.
2. Kshirsagar, R. et al. (2015). Clinical efficacy of Ksharasutra therapy in fistula-in-ano. Journal of Integrative Medicine.
3. Whitaker, I. S., & Rao, J. (2004). The role of leeches in plastic and reconstructive surgery. British Journal of Surgery.
4. Sharma, H., & Clark, C. (1998). Leech Therapy in Ayurveda and Modern Medicine. Lotus Press.

Ch. 8
Use of Ayurvedic Herbs for Pre- and Post-Operative Care

Ayurvedic herbs have been the cornerstone of healing in traditional medicine for thousands of years. Their incorporation into pre- and post-operative care optimizes patient outcomes by enhancing immune function, reducing inflammation, promoting tissue repair, and minimizing complications. This chapter explores the role of key Ayurvedic herbs and their formulations in surgical care, emphasizing their synergy with modern medicine.

Importance of Herbal Care in Surgery

Surgical procedures induce physiological stress, disrupt tissue integrity, and expose patients to risks of infection and delayed healing. Integrating Ayurvedic herbs provides:

- Immune modulation: Enhances the body's natural defense.
- Anti-inflammatory effects: Reduces swelling and pain.
- Antimicrobial properties: Prevents postoperative infections.
- Wound healing promotion: Stimulates regeneration and repair.
- Detoxification: Helps clear surgical toxins and metabolic wastes.

Preoperative Herbal Management

Preparing the patient before surgery is crucial for a smooth recovery. Ayurvedic preoperative care focuses on balancing the doshas, improving digestion (*Agni*), and detoxification.

- *Triphala*: A potent antioxidant blend of three fruits (*Amalaki*, *Bibhitaki*, *Haritaki*) that supports detoxification and bowel regulation.

- *Guduchi* (Tinospora cordifolia): Immunomodulator that enhances resistance and reduces inflammation.
- *Ashwagandha* (Withania somnifera): Adaptogen that reduces stress and improves stamina.
- Turmeric (Curcuma longa): Contains curcumin which prepares the body by reducing systemic inflammation.
- Usage: These herbs can be administered as powders, decoctions, or standardized extracts starting 1-2 weeks prior to surgery.

Postoperative Herbal Care

Post-surgery, the focus shifts to controlling pain, preventing infection, accelerating wound healing, and restoring strength. *Haridra* (Turmeric): Applied topically and consumed internally for its antimicrobial and anti-inflammatory effects.

- *Triphala Guggulu*: Supports detoxification and healing of surgical wounds.
- *Yashad Bhasma*: A traditional Ayurvedic zinc preparation that enhances tissue repair.
- *Madhuyasti* (Glycyrrhiza glabra): Anti-inflammatory and soothing for internal healing.
- *Jatyadi Taila*: An herbal oil widely used for external wound dressing, promoting rapid epithelialization and preventing infection.

Herbal Formulations and Dosage Forms

- Decoctions (Kwatha): Extract active phytochemicals, used for oral intake.
- Herbal Ghee (*Ghrita*): Enhances tissue nourishment and healing.
- Medicated Oils (*Taila*): Used for massage and wound dressing.
- Powders and Tablets: For easy administration and dose

standardization.

Scientific Evidence and Modern Insights

Numerous studies validate the efficacy of Ayurvedic herbs:

- Curcumin (from turmeric) modulates inflammatory pathways (NF-kB, COX-2 inhibition).
- *Guduchi* demonstrates immunomodulatory effects in clinical trials.
- *Triphala* exhibits antimicrobial and antioxidant properties beneficial in wound healing.
- *Jatyadi Taila* shows comparable wound healing effects to conventional topical agents.

Integrative Protocols in Surgical Practice

- Incorporate herbal supplements in pre-op clinics to reduce surgical stress.
- Use herbal oils and topical agents as adjuncts to standard wound care.
- Tailor herb selection based on patient constitution (*Prakriti*) and type of surgery.

References

1. Patwardhan, B., & Vaidya, A. D. B. (2010). Ayurveda and traditional Chinese medicine: A comparative overview. Evidence-Based Complementary and Alternative Medicine.
2. Aggarwal, B. B., & Harikumar, K. B. (2009). Potential therapeutic effects of curcumin, the anti-inflammatory agent, in cancer and chronic diseases. British Journal of Pharmacology.
3. Sharma, R., & Dash, B. (2001). Charaka Samhita. Chaukhamba Orientalia.
4. Singh, R. H. (2014). Herbal formulations in Ayurveda for wound healing. Journal of Ayurveda and Integrative Medicine.

Ch. 9
Ayurvedic Diet and Regimen for Surgical Patients

Optimal nutrition and lifestyle are fundamental pillars in Ayurveda for supporting the body's healing and regenerative capacities, particularly in surgical patients. An Ayurvedic diet tailored to individual constitution (*Prakriti*) and surgical requirements helps accelerate recovery, balance *Dosha*s, and restore vitality.

Importance of Diet in Surgical Recovery
Surgery creates physical trauma and metabolic stress, leading to increased nutritional demands. A proper diet:

- Supports tissue repair and regeneration
- Enhances immune response
- Reduces inflammation
- Prevents postoperative complications such as infection and delayed wound healing
- Restores digestive fire (*Agni*), crucial for nutrient assimilation

Principles of Ayurvedic Dietary Management
- *Dosha Bala*nce: Diet should correct any doshic im*Bala*nce caused by surgery or stress.
- Digestive Strength: Foods should be easy to digest, nourishing, and promote healthy *Agni*.
- Season and Environment: Dietary recommendations vary with seasons and climate.
- Patient's Constitution and Condition: Tailor food choices to individual needs and surgical type.

Preoperative Diet

Before surgery, the focus is on light, easily digestible foods that detoxify and prepare the body:

- Foods: Warm, cooked vegetables, rice, mung dal, light soups, herbal teas (ginger, cumin).
- Avoid: Heavy, oily, fried, or spicy foods that may aggravate *Pitta* or cause digestive sluggishness.
- Hydration: Warm water infused with herbs like coriander or fennel to maintain hydration and aid digestion.
- Herbs: Inclusion of *Trikatu* (black pepper, long pepper, ginger) to stimulate *Agni* gently.

Postoperative Diet

After surgery, the diet emphasizes healing and rebuilding tissue strength:

- Sattvic Foods: Fresh fruits, vegetables, whole grains, nuts, and dairy products like ghee and milk (if tolerated).
- Proteins: Mung dal, moong sprouts, and plant-based proteins help tissue repair.
- Herbal Supplements: Add *Rasayana*s (rejuvenatives) like *Ashwagandha* and A*Mala*ki to boost immunity.
- Soups and Broths: Nutritive, hydrating, and soothing for the digestive system.
- Avoid: Raw, cold, or heavy foods that burden digestion or increase *Kapha* leading to mucus and sluggishness.
- Meal Frequency: Small, frequent meals to prevent overloading the digestive system.

Regimen and Lifestyle Recommendations

- Rest and Sleep: Adequate rest enhances healing; Ayurveda emphasizes "*Diwaswapna*" (daytime rest) in early postoperative days.
- Gentle Exercise: Post-recovery, light yoga and breathing exercises help restore circulation and balance *Vata*.

- *Abhyanga* (Oil Massage): Mild massage with medicated oils improves circulation and calms the nervous system.
- Avoid Stress: Meditation and mindfulness practices reduce stress hormones detrimental to healing.

Sample Postoperative Ayurvedic Menu

Post-operative patients require:

- Energy ≈ 25-30 kcal/kg/day (↑ to 35 kcal/kg if major trauma / sepsis)
- Protein 1.2-2 g/kg/day (collagen, immune, nitrogen *Bala*nce)
- Adequate fluids & electrolytes (30 mL/kg/day baseline + losses)
- Micronutrients integral to wound repair – vit C (≥500 mg), Zn (15-30 mg), vit A, Cu, Se, arginine, glutamine

Ayurvedic view: surgery (śastra*karma*) aggravates *Vāta* (tissue injury, pain) and *Pitta* (inflammation). Diet should be:

- *Laghu* (light), *snigdha* (unctuous), *ushna* (warm) early on
- Progress via *Saṁsarjana Krama* – thin gruels → thicker → regular food as *Agni* (digestive capacity) returns
- Favour *Vāta-/Pitta-śāmaka* ingredients: moong, rice, ghee, cumin, ginger, turmeric, tender vegetables
- Avoid *guru* (heavy), *Kṣāra/amla* (very sour/fermented), *ati-kaṭu/tīkṣṇa* (very spicy), deep-fried

Core Nutritional Targets Mapped to Ayurvedic Vehicles

Modern Requirement	Ayurvedic-compatible Vehicle	Examples
Rapidly absorbable fluids & electrolytes	*Manda / yavāgu* (strained rice water), coconut water, coriander-cumin water	Na^+/K^+, hydration

Easily digestible protein	Moong yūṣa, thin dal, buttermilk (*takra*), soft-cooked eggs*, chicken bone broth*	*Non-veg optional
Quality fats (ω-3, SCFA precursor)	Cow ghee (1-2 tsp/meal), flaxseed powder, sesame oil (small qty)	Energy, SCFA, anti-inflammatory
Micronutrient boosters	Turmeric (curcumin), ginger, amla, carrot-beet broth	Antioxidant, vit C, β-carotene
Fiber for bowel recovery	Well-cooked vegetables (bottle gourd, zucchini, carrots), psyllium 3-5 g if opioid-induced constipation	Prevent ileus

Three-Day Sample Menu (Elective GI/General Surgery, Uncomplicated Course)

Day 0-1: Clear–Full Liquids (NPO until bowel sounds)

Time	Item	Volume	Rationale
06:00	Warm rice water (manda) + pinch saindhava (rock salt)	150 mL	Hydration, Na^+, laghu
09:00	Moong dal yūṣa (strained) with ½ tsp ghee	150 mL (6 g protein)	Easily digestible protein, SCFA
12:00	Tender coconut water (avoid if DM)	200 mL	Electrolytes, glucose
15:00	Ginger-cumin herbal tea	150 mL	Carminative, anti-emetic
18:00	Carrot-beet clear broth + turmeric pinch	150 mL	Antioxidant, carotenoids
21:00	Warm milk* + ½ tsp turmeric (golden milk)	150 mL	Tryptophan, curcumin

(*Lactose intolerant → almond milk)			

Day 2: Soft Semisolid (Peya/Vilepi Phase)

Meal	Menu	Nutritive Notes / kcal-protein
Breakfast	Rice-moong khichadi (1:1, pressure-cooked, 1 tsp ghee) + ½ cup stewed apple	350 kcal / 10 g
Mid-AM	Buttermilk (*takra*) with roasted cumin & coriander	Probiotic, 4 g
Lunch	Vegetable stew (bottle gourd, carrot, french beans) in thin coconut-milk base; soft red-rice idiyappam	400 kcal / 12 g
Snack	Roasted fox-nuts (makhana) lightly salted	Low-fat protein/ fiber
Dinner	Oats & moong dal porridge, tempered with ghee-ginger	300 kcal / 12 g
Bed-time	Warm chamomile-amla infusion	Vit C, sleep aid

Day 3-4: Transition to Regular (Akruta/Kruta)

Meal	Menu	kcal-protein
Breakfast	Ragi (finger millet) porridge with crushed peanuts, cardamom	Ca^{2+}, 12 g
Snack	5-6 soaked almonds + 1 date	150 kcal / 4 g
Lunch	Soft-chapati (whole wheat) + Palak-moong curry + ½ cup quinoa-vegetable pulao	500 kcal / 20 g
Evening	Turmeric-pepper chicken soup* OR tofu-spinach soup	150 kcal / 18 g
Dinner	Brown rice, sautéed zucchini & carrot, 1 cup curd	450 kcal / 14 g

*(*Omit animal protein for strict vegetarian patients)*

Expected totals: ~1,800-2,000 kcal, 80-90 g protein—modify for weight, catabolism, renal function.

Ingredient & Spice Notes

- Turmeric (500–1,000 mg curcumin/day) – anti-inflammatory, but watch peri-operative anticoagulation
- Ginger ≤2 g/day – pro-motility, anti-emetic, may ↑ bleeding risk in high doses
- Fenugreek seeds – glycemic control, but can cause bloating early
- Ghee – short-chain fatty acids (butyrate), use 3-4 tsp/day unless dyslipidemia
- Rock salt safer for gastritis than processed NaCl (lower sodium content disputed)

Red Flags / When to Hold or Modify Diet

- Persistent ileus, vomiting, new-onset abdominal pain – keep NPO, reassess anastomosis/leak
- Hyperglycemia >180 mg/dL – switch to low-GI carbs, regulate insulin
- eGFR <30 mL/min – restrict protein to 0.6-0.8 g/kg, avoid high K^+ foods (coconut water, bananas)
- Coumadin / DOAC – limit high-vit K greens, large turmeric/ginger doses
- Allergy to dairy, nuts, gluten – tailor substitutions

Monitoring & Follow-up

- Daily weight, fluid balance, serum electrolytes, glucose, albumin/prealbumin (trend)
- Wound inspection for dehiscence, SSI
- Bowel activity; add soluble fiber or laxatives if >48 h without flatus/stool
- Re-advance texture only after tolerance (no N+V, abdominal distension)

Patient-Facing Education Pearls (Lay Language)

"After your surgery, your digestive fire is weak, so we start with warm, light soups and thin rice water. Over three days we'll slowly thicken your meals, adding soft khichadi, vegetables, and gentle spices like ginger and turmeric that help reduce swelling and gas.

- Sip warm water; avoid iced drinks.
- Walk short distances to wake up your bowels.
- Skip fried or very spicy foods for at least a week.
- Call immediately if you have severe belly pain, fever, vomiting, or the wound looks red or leaks."

Scientific Correlation

- Studies show nutritional status significantly influences surgical outcomes.
- Ayurvedic emphasis on digestive fire corresponds to gut microbiome health, critical for immunity and recovery.
- Anti-inflammatory and antioxidant-rich foods in Ayurveda align with modern recommendations for postoperative care.

References

- ASPEN–SCCM Critical Care Nutrition Guidelines 2021 (evidence grade I)
    - ESPEN Post-operative Nutrition Guideline 2021
    - Sushruta Samhita, Chikitsa Sthana 1/44-55 (Saṁsarjana Krama)
    - NEJM 2022;387:135-147 – Enhanced Recovery After Surgery (ERAS) review
    - Curcumin meta-analysis on wound healing – Phytother Res 2022

1. Lad, V. (2002). Textbook of Ayurveda: Fundamental Principles. The Ayurvedic Press.

2. Bhattacharya, S. K. (2013). Nutritional aspects of Ayurveda and surgery. Journal of Clinical and Diagnostic Research.
3. Shankar, D., & Patwardhan, B. (2013). Integrative approaches to surgical nutrition. Evidence-Based Complementary and Alternative Medicine.

Ch. 10
Introduction to Laser Technology in Surgery

Laser technology represents one of the most significant advancements in modern surgical practice. Its precision, minimal invasiveness, and ability to target specific tissues have revolutionized how surgeons approach various medical conditions. This chapter introduces the fundamentals of laser technology, its types, mechanisms, and broad applications in surgery, setting the stage for its integration with traditional Ayurvedic principles.

What is a Laser?

The word LASER is an acronym for Light Amplification by Stimulated Emission of Radiation. A laser produces a concentrated beam of light that is:

- Monochromatic: Light of a single wavelength (color).
- Coherent: The light waves are in phase, resulting in a focused beam.
- Directional: Laser light travels in a narrow, precise path.
- Intense: It has a high degree of energy density, allowing for precise tissue interaction.

Principles of Laser Operation

Energy Source: The laser medium (gas, solid, liquid, or semiconductor) is energized (pumped) by an external energy source.

- Stimulated Emission: Excited atoms in the medium emit photons coherently.
- Amplification: These photons are amplified within a resonator cavity with mirrors reflecting light back and forth.

- Emission: A highly focused laser beam exits the device for clinical use.

Types of Surgical Lasers

Surgical lasers vary based on their active medium and wavelength, which determines their interaction with tissues:

- CO2 Laser: Emits infrared light, absorbed well by water in tissues; ideal for cutting and vaporizing soft tissue with minimal bleeding.
- Nd:YAG Laser: Penetrates deeper tissues, useful for coagulation and tumor ablation.
- Diode Laser: Compact, efficient, used widely in soft tissue surgeries including dental and proctology.
- Er:YAG Laser: High absorption by water, precise ablation with minimal thermal damage.

Mechanism of Laser-Tissue Interaction

Lasers affect tissue through various mechanisms:

- Photothermal: Heat generated by absorption of laser energy leads to vaporization or coagulation.
- Photochemical: Laser energy triggers chemical reactions (used in photodynamic therapy).
- Photoablation: Laser breaks molecular bonds, causing tissue removal without thermal damage.
- Photomechanical: High-energy pulses disrupt tissues mechanically.

Advantages of Laser Surgery

- Precision: Targets only diseased tissue sparing healthy structures.
- Minimal bleeding: Laser cauterizes blood vessels during cutting.
- Reduced pain and swelling: Less trauma leads to quicker recovery.

- Lower infection risk: Laser sterilizes the surgical field.
- Faster healing: Enhanced tissue repair post-procedure.
- Minimally invasive: Suitable for delicate and hard-to-reach areas.

Applications in Surgery

Lasers have broad applications including:

1. Dermatology: Removal of lesions, scars, and tattoos.
2. Ophthalmology: Corrective eye surgeries like LASIK.
3. ENT: Treatment of polyps, tonsillectomies.
4. Dentistry: Soft and hard tissue surgeries.
5. Proctology: Treatment of hemorrhoids, *fistulas*, and anal fissures.
6. Oncology: Tumor ablation and photodynamic therapy.

1. Fundamentals of Surgical Lasers

Laser = Light Amplification by Stimulated Emission of Radiation. Its key properties are:

- Monochromatic–single wavelength, allowing precise tissue targeting.
- Coherent–waves in phase, producing high energy density
- Collimated–minimal beam divergence, preserving focal accuracy.

Common Wavelengths & Chromophores

Wavelength	Absorption Target	Typical Use in Proctology
980 nm diode	Hemoglobin, water	Deep coagulation & hemorrhoidal shrinkage pubmed.ncbi.nlm.nih.gov
1,470 nm diode	Water	Superficial vaporization & ablation link.springer.com
10,600 nm CO_2	Water	Precise cutting & superficial tissue sculpting pubmed.ncbi.nlm.nih.gov

2. Mechanism of Action

Photothermal Effect

- Low power (5–15 W): Collagen contraction, vessel sealing → shrinkage of hemorrhoidal cushions or fistula tract lining link.springer.compubmed.ncbi.nlm.nih.gov
- High power (20–30 W): Vaporization and ablation of targeted tissue with minimal lateral thermal spread pubmed.ncbi.nlm.nih.gov

Selective Tissue Interaction

- Thin optical fibers (200–600 µm) are introduced into the submucosal plane or fistula tract, confining thermal injury.
- Surrounding healthy tissue remains intact when energy settings and withdrawal speed are respected pubmed.ncbi.nlm.nih.gov.

Delivery Modes

  - Continuous wave: Steady energy for smooth coagulation.
  - Pulsed mode: High peak power bursts for controlled ablation and minimized charring pubmed.ncbi.nlm.nih.gov.

3. Equipment & Safety

Laser Console: Variable power (5–30 W), continuous/pulsed settings, footswitch control.

Fibers & Handpieces:

- Radial emitting fibers for 360° energy distribution (FiLaC™).
- Straight fibers for pinpoint coagulation (LHP).

Safety Measures:

- *Manda*tory laser rated eyewear for all OR staff.
- Smoke evacuation to clear plume and reduce infective risk.

- Flame retardant drapes and avoidance of alcohol based prep solutions pubmed.ncbi.nlm.nih.gov.

4. Key Proctologic Procedures

4.1 Laser Hemorrhoidoplasty (LHP / LH)

Indications: Grade II–III symptomatic hemorrhoids.

Technique:

- Under anoscopic visualization, insert radial fiber into each hemorrhoidal cushion submucosally
- Deliver 6-8WAT in 1 second pulses while withdrawing fiber over 3–5 s.
- Coagulates submucosal vessels → gradual shrinkage of cushion.

Outcomes:

- Short term success: 98% stage reduction, low pain (VAS 0–1) by day 1 pubmed.ncbi.nlm.nih.gov.
- Long term recurrence: ~34% at 5 years (median 21 months) pubmed.ncbi.nlm.nih.gov.
- Meta analysis: ↓post op pain (MD –2.07 VAS units), ↓analgesia use, equivalent recurrence vs. open excision (HR 0.72) pmc.ncbi.nlm.nih.gov.

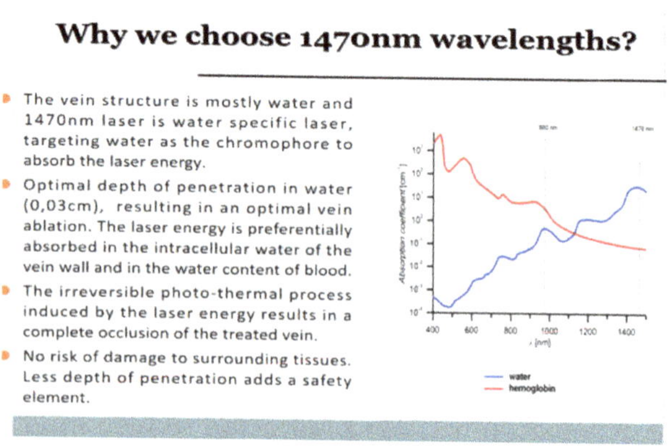

RESULTS OF LASER IN PROCTOLOGY

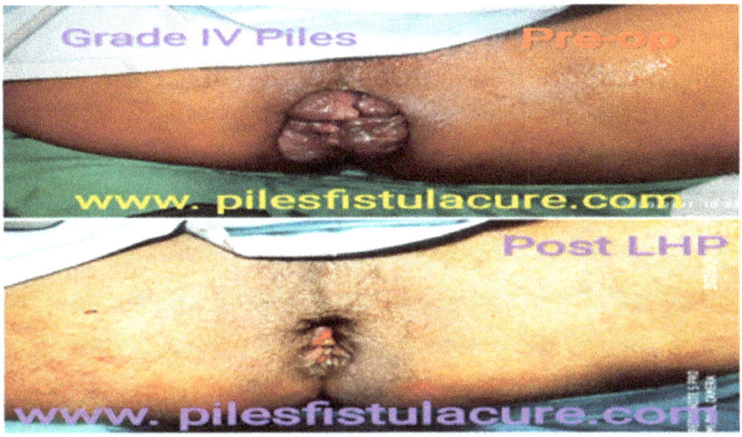

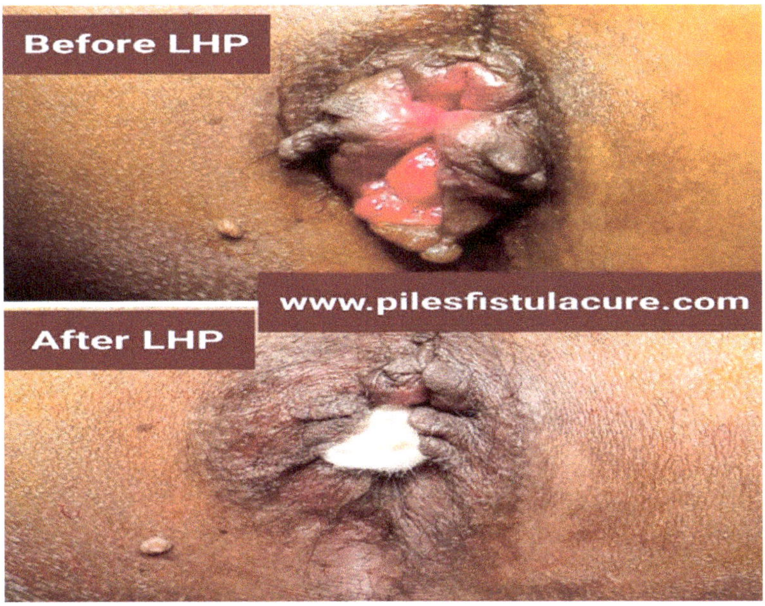

4.2 Fistula Laser Closure (FiLaC™)

Indications: Simple and complex cryptoglandular fistula in ano (trans and intersphincteric).

Technique:

- Map tract with probe/MRI; place seton if needed.
- Curette and irrigate to remove debris.
- Advance 360° radial fiber to internal opening.
- Withdraw at 1 mm/s with 10–12 W continuous power.

Outcomes:

- Primary healing: 63–67% (pooled) pubmed.ncbi.nlm.nih.govpubmed.ncbi.nlm.nih.gov.
- Secondary success (re FiLaC or adjunct): up to 88% link.springer.com.
- Complications: ~4–8% minor (abscess, minor incontinence) pubmed.ncbi.nlm.nih.gov.

FISTULA LASER RESULTS

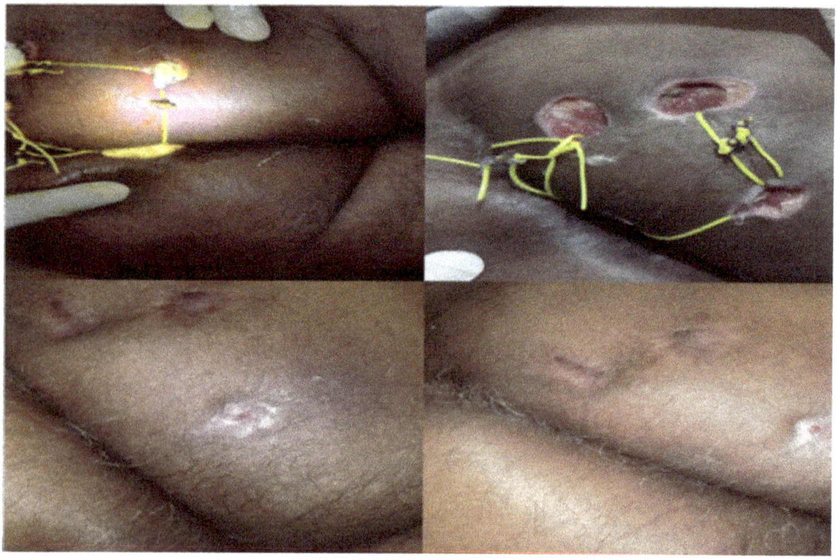

4.3 Laser Sphincterotomy for Anal Fissure

- Goal: Relieve internal sphincter spasm to promote fissure healing.
- Technique: Place fiber lateral to internal sphincter; apply 6–8 W continuous for 2–3 s.
- Benefits: Effective spasm relief with minimal collateral damage; data extrapolated from small series pubmed.ncbi.nlm.nih.gov.

4.4 Pilonidal Sinus Laser Ablation

- Indication: Uncomplicated pilonidal tracts.
- Technique: Fiber insertion into sinus, 10 W continuous energy in pulses → tract obliteration.
- Advantages: Outpatient, minimal scarring, rapid return to activity; evidence limited to case series pubmed.ncbi.nlm.nih.gov.

5. Clinical Workflow

- Preoperative: Full anorectal work up (anoscopy, endo anal ultrasound/MRI), bowel prep, prophylactic antibiotics.
- Anesthesia: Local ± sedation, or spinal block for patient comfort.
- Intraoperative: Continuous monitoring; precise fiber placement under direct vision.
- Postoperative:
    - Ambulatory discharge in 4–6 h (LHP, FiLaC).
    - Oral NSAIDs; sitz baths with *Triphala/Neem*.
    - Follow up at 1 wk and 1 mo for clinical assessment.

6. Advantages & Limitations

Advantages	Limitations
✓ Minimally invasive; no open excision	✗ Higher capital cost
✓ Bloodless field; excellent visibility	✗ Learning curve; requires specialized training
✓ Reduced postoperative pain & recovery	✗ Not ideal for extensive, branching fistulae
✓ Outpatient feasibility; quick return to work	✗ Long term recurrence (especially in LHP)

7. **Future Directions**

- AI guided dosimetry: Real time tissue feedback to adjust power.
- Ultra thin fibers & robotics: Access complex anatomy with micron precision.
- Hybrid techniques: Combining FiLaC with advancement flaps ↑primary success (95.5% vs. 72%) pubmed.ncbi.nlm.nih.gov.
- Robust RCTs: Needed to compare laser modalities head to head with other minimally invasive approaches.

Integrating Laser with Ayurveda

The precision and tissue-selective nature of lasers complement Ayurvedic principles of targeted healing and minimal intervention. Combining laser surgery with Ayurvedic herbal care can reduce complications, accelerate healing, and improve patient outcomes.

References

1. Sliney, D. H., & Menzel, H. G. (2000). Lasers in Surgery and Medicine: Principles and Applications. Springer.

2. Weiss, R. A., & McDaniel, D. H. (2014). The Art and Science of Laser Surgery. CRC Press.
3. Goldman, L. (2006). Lasers in Medicine and Surgery. McGraw-Hill.
4. Sharma, R. (2010). Ayurvedic principles in surgical laser application. Journal of Integrative Medicine.

Ch. 11
Physics and Principles of Surgical Lasers

Understanding the fundamental physics behind surgical lasers is essential for their safe and effective clinical application. This chapter delves into the physical properties of laser light, mechanisms of laser-tissue interaction, and the technical principles governing different types of surgical lasers.

Nature of Laser Light

Laser light possesses unique characteristics that differentiate it from ordinary light:

- Monochromaticity: Laser light consists of a single wavelength, producing a pure color and allowing precise targeting of tissues based on their absorption spectra.
- Coherence: The light waves are in phase both spatially and temporally, which enables the beam to be focused to a very small spot, enhancing precision.
- Directionality: Laser beams travel in parallel rays with minimal divergence, allowing surgeons to direct energy exactly where needed.
- High Intensity: Due to the concentration of photons, lasers deliver high energy density, enabling effective cutting, coagulation, or ablation.

Laser Medium and Types

Lasers are classified based on their active medium—the material that produces laser light when energized:

- Gas Lasers: CO_2 lasers (carbon dioxide) use a gas mixture and emit infrared light ideal for cutting soft tissues.

- Solid-State Lasers: Nd:YAG (neodymium-doped yttrium aluminum garnet) emit near-infrared light useful for coagulation and deep tissue pe*Netra*tion.
- Semiconductor (Diode) Lasers: Compact and versatile, used for soft tissue surgeries and proctological procedures.
- Liquid Lasers: Dye lasers that can be tuned to different wavelengths.

Laser-Tissue Interaction Mechanisms

When laser light strikes biological tissue, it can produce several effects depending on parameters like wavelength, power density, and exposure time:

- Absorption: Tissue chromophores (water, hemoglobin, melanin) absorb laser energy, converting it to heat.
- Reflection: Some light reflects off tissue surfaces and does not contribute to interaction.
- Transmission: Laser light passes through tissue if not absorbed.
- Scattering: Light may scatter within tissues, affecting the area of effect.

The absorbed energy causes:

- Photothermal Effects: Heat-induced coagulation, vaporization, or carbonization of tissue.
- Photochemical Effects: Initiation of chemical reactions, used in photodynamic therapy.
- Photoablation: Breaking molecular bonds to remove tissue without significant heat damage.
- Photomechanical Effects: High-energy pulses generate shockwaves that disrupt tissue mechanically.

Parameters Influencing Laser Surgery

1. Wavelength: Determines which chromophores absorb energy (e.g., water absorbs CO_2 laser; hemoglobin absorbs Nd:YAG).
2. Power Density (Irradiance): Higher power density increases tissue heating.
3. Exposure Time: Duration of laser application influences depth of tissue effect.
4. Pulse Mode: Continuous or pulsed lasers affect tissue differently; pulsed reduces thermal damage.

Laser Delivery Systems

- Handpieces and Fibers: Deliver laser light precisely to the surgical site.
- Focusing Lenses: Concentrate laser energy on a small spot.
- Cooling Systems: Protect adjacent tissues from heat damage.

Safety Considerations

1. Eye protection for patient and staff.
2. Proper training to avoid burns or unintended tissue damage.
3. Controlled environment to prevent laser reflections and accidents.

Clinical Implications

Understanding these principles allows surgeons to select the appropriate laser type and settings for each procedure, maximizing efficacy while minimizing complications. For example:

- CO_2 lasers for precise cutting with minimal bleeding.
- Nd:YAG lasers for deeper coagulation in vascular lesions.
- Diode lasers for soft tissue ablation with portability.

References

1. Sliney, D. H. (2016). Laser-tissue interactions: Fundamentals and clinical applications. Lasers in Surgery and Medicine, 48(9), 876-883.
2. Weiss, R. A., & McDaniel, D. H. (2014). The Art and Science of Laser Surgery. CRC Press.
3. Goldman, L. (2006). Lasers in Medicine and Surgery. McGraw-Hill.
4. Vogel, A., & Venugopalan, V. (2003). Mechanisms of pulsed laser ablation of biological tissues. Chemical Reviews, 103(2), 577-644.

Ch. 12
Common Anorectal Disorders: Hemorrhoids, Fissure In Ano , Fistula In Ano Pilonidal Sinus

Anorectal disorders are common conditions affecting millions worldwide, often causing significant discomfort and impacting quality of life. Understanding these disorders' pathology, symptoms, and treatment options—especially through integrative approaches combining Ayurveda and modern laser surgery—is crucial for effective management.

1. Hemorrhoids (Piles)

Definition:

Hemorrhoids are swollen vascular cushions in the anal canal. They become pathological when enlarged or inflamed, causing pain, bleeding, and discomfort.

Types:

- Internal Hemorrhoids: Located above the dentate line, usually painless but may cause bleeding.
- Grades of Internal hemorrhoids-

Grade I-Piles don't come outside only bleeding during defaecation.

Grade II-Piles comes while passing motion and reduce on their own.

Grade III-Piles comes during defaecation and needs to reduce it manually.

Grade IV-Piles remains outside and not reduceble .

- External Hemorrhoids: Below the dentate line, often painful and may thrombose.They are caused by inferior hemorrhoidal plexus.
- Mixed(External and Internal)hemorrhoids-They are resulting from anastomosis between inferior and surperior hemorrhoidal plexus.They may prolapse ,thrombosed or ulcerate.

Etiology:

There are different theories has been asumed since ancient times. Few accepted theories are as below

1. Sliding anal Cushion Theory: Thomson given the name to this theory of sliding anal cushion. Perianal connective tissue and conjoined longitudinal muscle are essential fibro-elastic elements that keep the anal cushions anchored.As the age progress the conestive tissue fibers around the blood vessels start to disintegrate and loosen and the veins become distended.Anal cushions are enlarged due to the hemorroidal tissue getting detached from he internal sphincter to slide down.In 1986 Goligher made the classification of internal hemorrhoids.
2. Hypervascularization Theory: Arterial blood supply of internal hemorrhoidal plexus is linked to hemorrhoid pathogenesis. The terminal branches of the superior hemorrhoidal artery supplying the anal cushions exhibited a three fold larger caliber, higher peak velocity, more blood flow and greater acceleration in hemorrhoids patients compared to healthy persons, resulting in hypervascularization.
3. Theory of straining and constipation: Burkitt elaborated low fiber diet s a cause of hemorrhoid.Constipation is increased by repeated and prolonged straining while passing hard stools causing hemorrhoid prolapse.

Low fiber dier

↓

Less bulky stool

↓

straining at defaecation

↓

Increased intra-anal pressure

↓

Decreased venous return

↓

Enlarged anal cushion

↓

Hemorrhoids

Common Causes of Hemorrhoids:

- Chronic Constipation or Straining:

Straining during bowel movements increases pressure on rectal veins.Hard stools can irritate or damage the anal canal.

- Prolonged Sitting (especially on the toilet):

This can cause blood to pool in the anal area, leading to vein swelling.

- ***Low-Fiber Diet:***

A diet lacking in fiber leads to harder stools and constipation.

- ***Obesity***

Excess weight increases abdominal pressure, stressing pelvic veins

- ***Pregnancy***

The growing uterus compresses veins, and hormonal changes cause vein dilation.Common especially in the third trimester.

- ***Chronic Diarrhea:***

Frequent bowel movements can irritate and inflame the rectal area.

- ***Heavy Lifting:***

Regularly lifting heavy weights increases intra-abdominal pressure.

- ***Aging***:

Tissues supporting rectal veins weaken with age, making hemorrhoids more likely.

- ***Genetic Predisposition:***

A family history of hemorrhoids may increase individual risk.

- ***Portal Hypertension (in some cases):***

Increased pressure in the portal vein system usually due to liver cirrhosis leading to the formation of portosystemic collaterals.

- **Symptoms:**

1. Bleeding:

Bright red and painless bleeding in the form of dripping in the toilet,spurt or wipping with tissue paper after defaecation .

2. Prolapse:

Internal piles classified depending on the degree of prolapse

Grade I-Piles don't come outside only bleeding during defaecation.

Grade II-Piles comes while passing motion and reduce on their own.

Grade III-Piles comes during defaecation and needs to reduce it manually.

Grade IV-Piles remains outside and not reducible.

3. *Thrombosis:*
The whole part of hemorrhoid become swollen along with anal cushion and become thrombosed.

4. *Musus discharge:*
The columnar mucosa extend beyond the anal canal leads to irritation ,itching at anal region and mucus secreation.

5. *Pain:*
Bleeding, extreme pain, swelling at anal mucosa is suggesting strangulated hemorrhoid pile mass

- ***Ayurvedic Perspective:***

Certainly. Hemorrhoids (known as *Arsha* or अर्शः in Sanskrit) are thoroughly discussed in the classical Ayurvedic texts—*Charaka Samhita*, *Sushruta Samhita*, and *Ashtanga Hridaya* by *Vagbhata*.

Below is a structured summary of the causes, types, and Ayurvedic understanding of hemorrhoids (*Arsha*) according to these classical texts, along with relevant *Sanskrit shlokas*:

1. Definition of Arsha (Hemorrhoids)

Sushruta Samhita - Nidana Sthana 6.3

"अर्शो नाम व्याधिरनुपहतोऽप्यतिरुजः स्यात् ।"

Arśo nāma vyādhir anupahato'py atirujaḥ syāt.

Translation: *Arsha* is a disease which, even without direct injury, causes severe pain.

2. Causes of Arsha (Hemorrhoids)

Common Causes as per All Three Texts:

1. Consumption of excessively heavy, dry, spicy, or incompatible foods.
2. Excessive sitting or sedentary lifestyle.
3. Suppression of natural urges (*Vegadharana*).
4. Overeating or indigestion (*Ajeerna*).
5. Excessive sexual activity.
6. Constipation or straining during defecation.

Charaka Samhita - Chikitsa Sthana 14.5-6

"आतपशीतवातात्युद्वर्तनगमनासनैः ।
व्यायामशय्यातिव्यवायभोजनविसर्जनैः ।।५।।
पाचनं दीपनोद्दीप्यं विदाहिजननं तथा ।
रूक्षं तिक्तं कषायं च कटु चाम्लं च सेवतः ।।६।।"

Following are the causes of arsha disease-

- Excessive exposure to sun, cold wind
- Friction (rubbing), walking, sitting, exercise
- Sleeping during the day,
- Excessive sex,
- Untimely eating or excretion, consumption of pungent, sour, rough, bitter, and astringent food, and food that causes burning sensation and indigestion

7. Sushruta Samhita - Nidana Sthana 6.5

"कृशानां स्निग्धदुष्टानां रूक्षभोजनसेविनाम् ।
अनाहारिणां चात्यर्थं स्यातां वातकफार्शसि ।।५।।"

Those who are emaciated, consume spoiled oily food, take dry food, or stay on an empty stomach for long may develop *Vata-Kapha* type *Arsha*.

3. Dosha-Based Classification of Arsha

As per *Tridosha* theory, *Arsha* is classified into:

1. *Vata*ja *Arsha* (dry, painful, fissure-like)
2. *Pitta*ja *Arsha* (burning, bleeding, inflamed)
3. *Kapha*ja *Arsha* (soft, pale, non-painful)
4. Sannipataja *Arsha* (mixed *Dosha*s, severe)
5. *Raktaja Arsha* (bleeding type, linked with blood vitiation)
6. *Sahaja Arsha* (hereditary, present since birth)

- *Ashtanga Hridaya - Nidana Sthana* 8.1-3

  "कटुकोष्णाम्ललवणं तिक्तं रूक्षं कषायकम्।
  गुरु चाम्लं च भोजनं मात्रा त्यक्त्वा च भुज्यते।।१।।
  ...तेषां पाचनदीपनैर्विशेषेण विधीयते।
  त्रिदोषकृतमेवाहुर्नानात्मजमिति स्थितिः।।३।।"

Foods that are pungent, hot, sour, bitter, dry, astringent, heavy, or acidic in excess disturb the Balance of *dosha*s and are considered causative of *Arsha*. *Arsha* is mostly caused by the three *dosha*s (*Vata*, *Pitta*, *Kapha*).

4. Types of Arsha

- According to Origin (*Samprapti*):

1. *Sadhya Arsha* – Curable
2. *Yapya Arsha* – Manageable but not curable
3. *Asadhya Arsha* – Incurable (due to genetic factors or severe doshic involvement)

- *Sushruta Samhita - Chikitsa Sthana* 6.3

  "अरिशोभेदं त्रिविधं सम्प्रधार्यं नराधिप।
  साध्यमुपशयं चैव याप्यं चोपलक्षयेत्।।"

The types of hemorrhoids are to be recognized as curable (*Sadhya*), palliable (*Yapya*), or incurable (*asadhya*).

5. Summary of Ayurvedic View

Concept	Detail
Name	*Arsha* (अर्शः)
Cause (*Nidana*)	Improper diet, sedentary life, suppression of urges, overexertion
Doshas Involved	*Vata, Pitta, Kapha* – individually or combined
Site	*Guda* (anus/rectum)
Types	*Vataja, Pittaja, Kaphaja, Tridoshaja, Raktaja, Sahaja*
Symptoms	Pain, bleeding, swelling, itching, burning, prolapse (in advanced)

Ayurveda, particularly through the classical texts like *Sushruta Samhita*, *Charaka Samhita*, and *Ashtanga Hridaya* (by *Vagbhata*), offers detailed descriptions and surgical principles for treating *Arsha* (अर्शः) — the Ayurvedic term for hemorrhoids or piles. Below is a consolidated overview of the surgical principles of hemorrhoid treatment as described in these texts, with relevant S*anskrit shlokas*:

1. Surgical Principles from Sushruta Samhita

Sushruta, known as the father of surgery, provides the most elaborate surgical description of hemorrhoids in the *Nidana Sthana* and *Chikitsa Sthana.*

- Surgical Treatments (for *Arsha*):
    - *Kshara Karma* (Cauterization with alkaline paste)
    - *Agni Karma* (Thermal cauterization)
    - *Shastra Karma* (Surgical excision)

A. *Shastra Karma* (Surgical Excision)

श्लोक (*Sushruta Samhita*, *Chikitsa Sthana*, Chapter 6.15–17):

"तेषां त्रिविधं कर्म स्यादर्शसां शस्त्रकषाराग्निभिः।
स्निग्धोष्णवस्त्रसंवीतान् बद्धाङ्गुलिसमाहतात।।
शस्त्रेण तु विशेषेण सम्पूर्णान् मूलतः क्षिपेत्।
संस्पृशेदग्निना पश्चात् क्षारद्रव्यं न तु क्षिपेत्।।"

There are three main treatments for hemorrhoids: *shastra* (surgery), *kshara* (alkaline cautery), and *Agni* (thermal cautery). Fully formed piles should be removed surgically and then cauterized to prevent recurrence.

B. *Kshara Karma* (Chemical cauterization):

Sushruta Samhita, *Chikitsa Sthana*, 6.24–25:

"असाराणि तु दारुण्यान्यथाऽर्शांसि सुलक्षणान्।
क्षारद्रव्येण संदग्ध्वा व्रणं पाययितं हितम्।।"

In cases where piles are hard and chronic, application of alkaline substances (*Kshara*) is recommended to destroy them, followed by wound healing protocols.

C. *Agni Karma* (Thermal cauterization):

"येषां शस्त्रकषारेण न सिद्धिर्भवति ध्रुवम्।
तत्राग्निकर्म कर्तव्यमर्शोभ्यस्तानि पूरयेत्।।"

In cases where *Shastra* or *Kshara* treatment is not effective, thermal cauterization should be done.

2. *Charaka Samhita* on *Arsh*a (Non-surgical emphasis)

Charaka primarily emphasizes internal medicine but acknowledges surgical methods for external hemorrhoids.

"येषां चोपशमं नायाति भेषजैरपि सर्वशः।
तेषां यथोक्तं कर्म कुर्यादर्शो विनाशनम्।।"

(*Charaka Chikitsa Sthana*, Chapter 14.32):

When medicinal treatments do not provide relief in piles, the appropriate surgical procedures should be adopted to eliminate them.

3. *Vagbhata – Ashtanga Hridaya*

Vagbhata synthesizes *Sushruta* and *Charaka*'s views.

"कषारेण तु दग्ध्वाऽथ वह्निना चोपशोषयेत् ।
नास्त्यग्निकर्मसममर्शोघ्नं किञ्चिद् इह औषधम् ।।"

(*Ashtanga Hridaya*, *Chikitsa Sthana*, *Arsha Chikitsa*, 8.25–26)

Kshara or *Agni* should be used to cauterize hemorrhoids; there is no treatment as effective as *Agni Karma* in eliminating piles.

Summary Table

Text	**Treatment Modalities**	**Key Principle**
Sushruta Samhita	*Shastra, Kshara, Agni Karma*	Surgical focus
Charaka Samhita	*Bheshaja (Medicines), then Shastra if needed*	Internal first
Ashtanga Hridaya	*Kshara, Agni; rarely Shastra*	Combined approach

Post-operative Care (*Sushruta*):

Use of Sitz bath (*Avagaha Sweda*)

Herbal fumigation (*Dhoomapana*)

Application of wound-healing herbs like *Jatyadi Ghrita*, *Ropan Taila*

Modern Treatment of Hemorrhoids: ASCRS Guidelines (2024)

1. Evaluation and Diagnosis

The American Society of Colon and Rectal Surgeons (ASCRS)

emphasizes a detailed clinical history and physical examination as the cornerstone of hemorrhoid evaluation. In patients presenting with rectal bleeding, a full colon evaluation, including colonoscopy, is advised to rule out colorectal neoplasia.

2. *First-Line: Lifestyle and Medical Therapy*

High-fiber diet (20–35 g/day), increased water intake, and avoidance of straining are key recommendations. Medical therapy includes:

- Bulk-forming laxatives
- Topical corticosteroids
- Local anesthetics (e.g., lidocaine)
- Astringents (e.g., witch hazel)
- Venoactive agents (e.g., MPFF)

3. *Office-Based (Outpatient) Procedures*

These are preferred for Grade I–II and selected Grade III internal hemorrhoids:

- Rubber Band Ligation (RBL): First-line office procedure
- Sclerotherapy: Safe in anticoagulated patients
- Infrared Coagulation (IRC): Non-invasive but may require multiple sessions

4. *Surgical Treatment*

Indicated for Grade III–IV, thrombosed, or refractory hemorrhoids:

- Excisional Hemorrhoidectomy (Milligan-Morgan/Ferguson): Most effective for advanced disease
- Doppler-Guided Hemorrhoid Artery Ligation (DG-HAL): Less painful, higher recurrence
- Stapled Hemorrhoidopexy (PPH): Not routinely recommended
- Thrombosed External Hemorrhoids: Surgical excision within 72 hours

5. Special Considerations

Immunocompromised patients should be treated conservatively. If procedures are needed, a cautious approach with preference for non-excisional methods is recommended.

6. Summary of Treatment Recommendations (ASCRS)

Clinical Scenario	**Recommended Treatment**
Symptomatic Grades I–II	Lifestyle + fiber + medical therapy ± office procedures
Refractory Grade III	RBL; if ineffective, consider DG-HAL or excisional hemorrhoidectomy
Grade IV / External / Mixed Hemorrhoids	Excisional hemorrhoidectomy
Thrombosed External Hemorrhoid (within 4 days)	Early surgical excision
Immunocompromised	Conservative management preferred; interventions used cautiously

Reference -ASCRS 2024 guidelines (Hawkins et al., Dis Colon Rectum) and guideline summaries from gastroenterology advisor & Medscape.

Laser Hemorrhoidoplasty (LHP): Clinical Application and Research Evidence

1. Introduction

Laser Hemorrhoidoplasty (LHP) is a minimally invasive surgical procedure that uses laser energy to obliterate internal hemorrhoids by reducing blood supply and inducing fibrosis. It is particularly effective in Grades II–III hemorrhoids and has emerged as a popular alternative to conventional hemorrhoidectomy due to its reduced pain and faster recovery.

2. *Clinical Evidence Summary*

Numerous clinical studies have validated LHP as a safe and effective treatment. A Bangladeshi study on 86 patients reported 100% reduction in hemorrhoid size and 97.7% patient satisfaction. Complications were low and manageable.

Comparative trials with LigaSure and open hemorrhoidectomy consistently showed:

- Lower postoperative pain (VAS score 1–2)
- Shorter operative times (15–20 minutes)
- Faster return to work (within 2–7 days)
- Slightly higher recurrence (up to 22% in some cohorts)

Enhanced techniques combining LHP with mucopexy or blind artery ligation have shown superior results.

3. *Long-Term Outcomes*

A prospective cohort from Faridpur Medical College followed 100 patients for 3 years, demonstrating:

- Low recurrence (2%)
- Quick return to normal life
- Minimal complications

Other trials across Asia and Europe confirm LHP as a durable option for managing hemorrhoids with favorable patient outcomes.

4. *Summary Table: LHP vs Conventional Surgery*

Feature	Laser Hemorrhoidoplasty (LHP)	Conventional Surgery
Operative Time	~15–18 min	~25–30 min
Postoperative Pain	Low (VAS 1–2)	High (VAS 5–7)

Return to Normal Life	2–7 days	5–14 days
Complications	Minor (<20%)	Moderate (~30–40%)
Recurrence (1 year)	2–22%	6–10%
Long-Term Recurrence	~2% (3 years)	Similar or lower

5. ***Patient Perspectives***

Patients report minimal pain post-procedure and rapid recovery. However, rare complications such as fissures, serous discharge, or minor bleeding have been noted. Most agree LHP is preferable over traditional hemorrhoidectomy.

6. ***Practical Considerations for LHP fits well into modern hemorrhoid management as a minimally invasive alternative that can be offered in outpatient settings.***

Laser Hemorrhoidoplasty (LHP): A Comprehensive Book Chapter

1. ***Mechanism and Rationale of LHP***

Laser Hemorrhoidoplasty (LHP) uses a diode laser (commonly 980–1470 nm wavelength) to deliver controlled thermal energy into the submucosal hemorrhoidal plexus. The energy denatures proteins, causes endothelial coagulation, and reduces blood flow, leading to shrinkage and fibrosis of the hemorrhoidal tissue without excising the mucosa. This minimally invasive approach minimizes postoperative pain and preserves anatomical integrity.

2. ***Evidence from RCTs and Cohort Studies***

Clinical evidence from randomized controlled trials and cohort studies highlights the effectiveness and safety of LHP:

- A Bangladeshi prospective study (2023) with 86 patients

(mostly Grade III) demonstrated 100% size reduction and 97.7% satisfaction.

- Kosovo RCT (2022) comparing LHP with open hemorrhoidectomy found significantly lower pain and faster recovery in the LHP group.
- Meta-analysis (2023) concluded LHP is associated with lower postoperative pain and faster return to work compared to excisional techniques.
- Long-term follow-up from Faridpur Medical College (3 years) showed only 2% recurrence with minimal complications.

3. *Comparative Benefits and Drawbacks*

Benefits:

- Minimally invasive
- Reduced postoperative pain
- Shorter operative time
- Quicker return to normal activities
- Suitable for outpatient setting

Drawbacks:

- Slightly higher recurrence in some studies (especially without mucopexy)
- Requires laser equipment and training
- Potential complications: fissure, bleeding, seroma

4. *Role in Advanced Hemorrhoids (LHP + Ligation/Mucopexy)*

In Grades III–IV hemorrhoids, LHP alone may be insufficient. Combining it with:

- Blind or Doppler-guided arterial ligation enhances dearterialization.
- Mucopexy tacks prolapsed tissue back into the anal canal.
- This hybrid approach improves anatomical and symptomatic outcomes and reduces recurrence.

5. Diagram & Flowchart (Visual Aid)

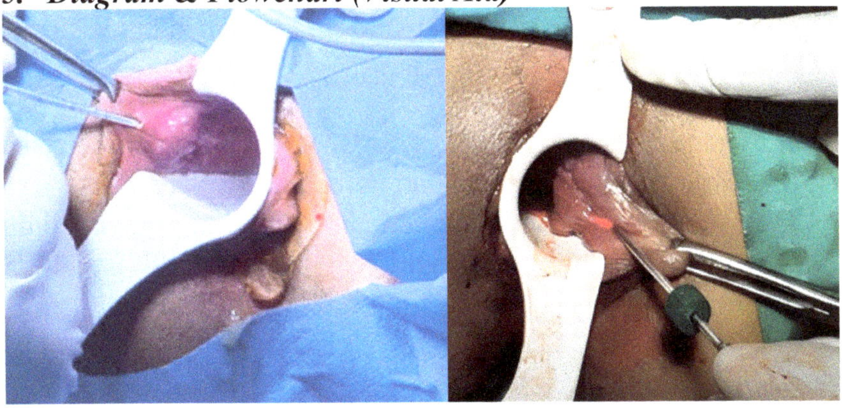

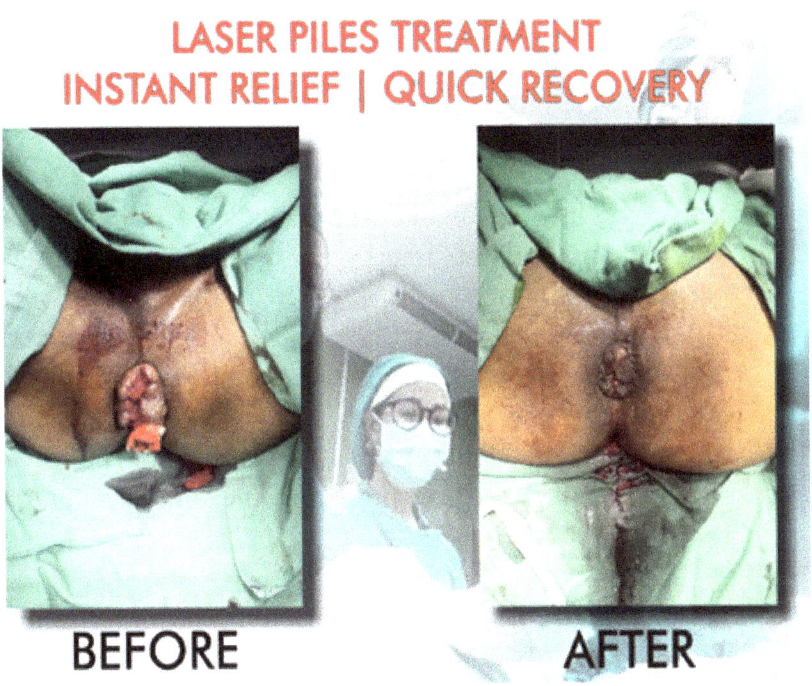

Laser Energy Application Pathway

The laser energy application pathway refers to the systematic route through which laser energy is delivered and absorbed by biological tissues during a surgical or therapeutic procedure.

Understanding this pathway is crucial for optimizing treatment outcomes, minimizing tissue damage, and enhancing precision.

1. Laser Generation

- Lasers such as CO_2, diode, Er:YAG, and Nd:YAG are selected based on their wavelength and tissue affinity.
- The laser system converts electrical energy into coherent light energy at specific wavelengths (e.g., 810 nm, 980 nm, 1470 nm).

2. Delivery System

- Laser energy is typically delivered through:
  - Optical fibers (flexible glass fibers for endoscopic use)
  - Handpieces (for external or superficial treatment)
  - Articulated arms (commonly in CO_2 lasers)

3. Tissue Interaction

- Laser energy interacts with tissue through:
  - Photothermal effect: Energy converts to heat, cutting or coagulating tissue.
  - Photomechanical effect: Shockwaves for tissue disruption.
  - Photochemical effect: Stimulates biological changes at the cellular level.
- Each wavelength determines depth of pe*Netra*tion and absorption (e.g., water, hemoglobin, melanin are common chromophores).

4. Targeted Action

- Laser energy is directed toward specific pathology:
  - Hemorrhoidal tissue (causing shrinkage)
  - Fistula tracts (ablation)
  - Anal polyps or skin tags (vaporization)

5. ***Feedback & Control***

- Modern systems allow:
  - Real-time feedback for temperature and energy output
  - Preset modes for cutting, coagulation, or ablation
  - Safety features like pulse modulation and shut-off sensors

6. ***Tissue Response & Healing***

- Proper application ensures:
  - Minimal collateral damage
  - Reduced bleeding and inflammation
  - Faster epithelial regeneration and wound closure

- Comparison of LHP vs. traditional hemorrhoidectomy

LHP (Laser Hemorrhoidoplasty) vs. Traditional Hemorrhoidectomy

Aspect	**LHP (Laser Hemorrhoido-plasty)**	**Traditional Hemor-rhoidectomy**
Technique	Minimally invasive laser coagulation of hemorrhoidal tissue	Excision of hemorrhoids with scalpel/electrocau-tery
Anesthesia	Usually local or regional anesthesia	Typically requires spinal or general anesthesia
Pain (Post-operative)	Mild to minimal discomfort	Moderate to severe pain due to open wounds
Bleeding	Very minimal (coagulative laser effect seals vessels)	Moderate to significant (risk during and after surgery)
Wound	No open wound; intact ano-derm	Open wound at the sur-gical site
Healing Time	Faster (5–7 days average)	Longer (2–4 weeks)
Hospital Stay	Often daycare or short stay (few hours)	Often requires overnight hospitalization

Recurrence Rate	Comparable or slightly lower with proper technique	Low, but potential scarring and stenosis risk
Return to Work/Activity	2–3 days (depends on severity and occupation)	7–14 days or more
Complications	Rare: minimal infection, no anal stenosis	Possible: anal stenosis, incontinence, delayed healing
Cosmetic Outcome	Excellent (no visible scars)	Poorer (visible scarring, sometimes deformity)
Cost	Higher (due to laser equipment cost)	Lower upfront cost

Conclusion:

- LHP offers a safer, less painful, and cosmetically superior alternative, especially in Grade II–III hemorrhoids.
- Traditional hemorrhoidectomy remains the gold standard in severe (Grade IV) or complicated cases, but involves more postoperative morbidity.

Decision-Making Algorithm for Grade I–IV Hemorrhoids

Step 1: Clinical Assessment

- History: Bleeding, prolapse, pain, discharge, itching.
- Physical exam: Digital rectal exam (DRE), anoscopy/proctoscopy.
- Grade classification (Goligher's classification):

Grade	Description
I	Bleeding only, no prolapse
II	Prolapse with spontaneous reduction
III	Prolapse requiring manual reduction
IV	Irreducible prolapse

Step 2: Treatment Decision Tree

Grade I

- Conservative Management
    - High-fiber diet, hydration
    - Sitz baths, topical creams
    - Flavonoids (Daflon, etc.)

- If unresponsive → Outpatient procedures
    - Rubber band ligation (RBL)
    - Infrared coagulation (IRC)

Grade II

- Office-based Interventions First
    - RBL / IRC / Sclerotherapy
- If symptomatic recurrence → LHP or Doppler-guided hemorrhoidal artery ligation (DG-HAL)

Grade III

- Depends on tissue quality and patient preference
    - LHP: Ideal for patients desiring fast recovery, minimal pain
    - DG-HAL/RAR (Recto-anal repair): Effective for bulging hemorrhoids
    - Conventional hemorrhoidectomy: If fibrotic, large, or irreducible

Grade IV

- Surgical Approach Required
    - Conventional open/closed hemorrhoidectomy
    - LHP as adjunct in select, localized cases with less prolapse
    - Stapled hemorrhoidopexy (Longo) in suitable case

Additional Considerations

- Patient factors: Age, comorbidities, occupation, pain tolerance.
- Anesthesia preference: LHP = local/regional; traditional = spinal/general.
- Recurrence history: Recurrent cases may favor LHP or surgical intervention.
- Cost and availability: Laser equipment and expertise may vary by region.

6. Patient FAQs

Q1. Is laser hemorrhoid surgery painful?

A1. It is significantly less painful than traditional surgery.

Q2. How long does recovery take?

A2. Most patients return to normal activity in 2–7 days.

Q3. Are the hemorrhoids permanently removed?

A3. The hemorrhoids shrink and fibrose. There is a small chance of recurrence (2–22% depending on grade).

Q4. Is it done under general anesthesia?

A4. Often performed under local, regional, or short general anesthesia.

Q5. Are there any complications?

A5. Rarely, patients may develop serous discharge, minor bleeding, or anal fissures.

Anal Fissures & Laser Sphincterotomy

1. Micro Anatomy & Pathophysiology

Anoderm & Dentate Line

The fissure typically involves the anoderm distal to the dentate line, supplied by somatic inferior rectal nerves → excruciating pain on defecation.

Internal Anal Sphincter (IAS)

70% of resting pressure; chronic hypertonia → reduced anodermal perfusion → ischemia → failure to heal.

Ischemia Spasm Pain Cycle

Pain → sphincter spasm

Spasm → decreased blood flow

Ischemia → non healing fissure

Interrupting this cycle is the key therapeutic goal.

2. *Laser Physics & Tissue Interaction*

Choice of Wavelength

- Diode 980 nm: *Bala*nced absorption in hemoglobin and water; penetration ~2–3 mm.
- Diode 1,470 nm: High water absorption; shallow effect (~1 mm), ideal for surface ablation.
- CO_2 (10,600 nm): Very high water absorption; ultra precise superficial vaporization.

Energy Density (Fluence)

- Expressed as J/cm^2; governs depth of coagulation vs. ablation.

Power & Mode

- Continuous Wave (CW): Steady output, consistent thermal effect.
- Pulsed Mode: High peak power pulses with inter pulse cooling, limits lateral thermal spread.

3. *Patient Selection & Contraindications*

Ideal Candidates

- Chronic (>6 weeks), non healing fissures refractory to maximal topical and injectable therapies.
- Patients with high surgical risk for incontinence (multiparous women, elderly).

Contraindications

- Acute fissure (<6 weeks) that may heal with conservative care.
- Coexisting anorectal sepsis or complex anal fistula.
- Severe anal stenosis or Crohn's disease active lesions.

4. *Pre Operative Protocol*

History & Examination

- Document fissure duration, pain scale (VAS), prior treatments.
- Rule out secondary causes: IBD, neoplasm.

Imaging

- Endo anal ultrasound or MRI if suspicion of secondary fistula or sepsis.

Bowel Preparation

- Low residue diet 24 h pre op; fleet enema on morning of surgery.

Informed Consent

- Discuss sphincter sparing nature, expected healing timeline, possible need for repeat session.

5. *Laser Sphincterotomy Technique*

5.1 Equipment Setup

Laser Console: Set to 10 W CW (diode) or 15 W CW (CO_2 fractional).

Handpiece & Fiber: 400 μm radial fiber tip for uniform coverage.

Monitoring: Pulse oximeter, ECG, non invasive BP.

5.2 Patient Positioning & Anesthesia

Position: Prone jack knife or lithotomy.

Anesthesia:

Local Infiltration: 0.5% bupivacaine around fissure edges.

Sedation: IV midazolam/fentanyl for comfort.

Optional: Spinal block for anxious patients.

5.3 Step by Step Procedure

Exposure

Retract buttocks; gently dilate anal verge with small lubricated speculum.

Assessment

Inspect fissure bed, hypertrophied papillae, sentinel pile.

Laser Application

Non contact mode: Position fiber 1–2 mm from tissue surface.

Infiltrate 2 ml of Lox with adrenalin solution at mucosa at 5 o clock at anal region to elevate mucosa from Internal sphincter Insert Laser Bare fiber from mucosa to internal sphincter and cut internal sphincter fiber. Press for few minutes and apply ice cubes.

Another method is to cut internal sphincter from interspchencteric groove at 5 o clock position.Press for few minutes and apply icecubes.

Coverage:

First pass: entire fissure length at 1 cm intervals.

Second pass: edges and base with overlapping spots.

Energy Delivery:
Diode 980 nm @ 10 W CW, 2 s per spot (≈ 20 J/spot).

CO_2 fractional @15 W continuous, 3–5 passes to depth ~3–4 mm.

Hemostasis Check
Observe for immediate blanching and mild contraction; no bleeding expected.

Dressing
Apply a thin layer of *Jatyadi Taila* or antibiotic ointment; no sutures.

6. Post Op Care & Rehabilitation

Immediate
- Monitor in recovery for 30 min; vital signs stable → discharge.

Medications
- Analgesics: NSAIDs (e.g. ibuprofen) for 3 days.
- Stool Softeners: Polyethylene glycol for 1 week.

Local Care
- Sitz Baths: Warm water 2–3×/day with *Triphala* decoction.
- Topicals: Turmeric *Guggulu* paste applied to fissure site.

Follow Up
- Week 1: Wound check; pain assessment, ensure no infection.
- Week 4: Evaluate fissure closure; assess for hypertrophic papilla resolution.

7. *Outcomes & Evidence*

Metric	Laser Sphincterotomy	Lateral Internal Sphincterotomy (LIS)
Healing Rate	90–100% at 3 mo	~95% at 3 mo
Post Op Pain (VAS)	0–2 (day 1)	3–5 (day 1)
Incontinence Risk	< 1%	10–15% (minor flatus/ fecal incontinence)
Return to Work	1–2 days	7–10 days
Recurrence	~5–10%	~5%

Data synthesized from CO_2 and diode laser series (Esfahani 2015; Fateh 2016; Pappas 2017).

8. *Complications & Management*

Transient Bleeding (< 5%)

- Apply direct pressure; rarely require cautery.

Local Infection (< 3%)

- Oral antibiotics; ensure adequate sitz baths.

Thermal Injury of IAS (> 2%)

- Prevent by strict adherence to power/duration; managed conservatively.

Persistent Fissure/Non Healing (5–10%)

- Repeat laser session or consider partial LIS

9. *Future Research & Innovations*

Dose Response Studies

Optimal fluence and pulse vs. CW modes for maximal efficacy with zero collateral damage.

Real Time Tissue Feedback
Optical coherence tomography (OCT) probes integrated into fiber tips.

Combination Therapies
Laser + topical stem cell therapy or platelet rich plasma to further accelerate mucosal regeneration.

Randomized Trials
Head to head comparisons with LIS in large multicenter cohorts to establish Level I evidence.

10. Illustrations & Diagrams to Include

Microanatomy of the Internal Anal Sphincter (IAS)

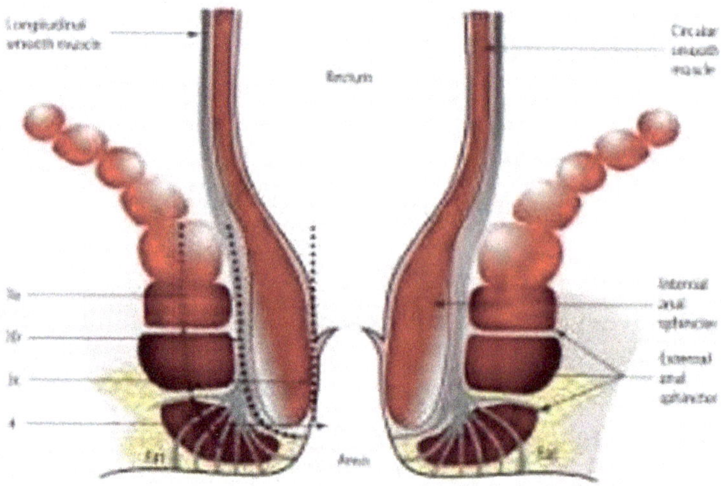

1. Layers (from inside out):

Mucosa

- Lined by columnar epithelium (upper anal canal), transitioning to stratified squamous non-keratinized epithelium and finally to keratinized skin (at the anal verge).
- Contains anal columns, crypts, and anal glands.

Submucosa

Contains connective tissue, blood vessels, lymphatics, and glands.

Internal Anal Sphincter (IAS)

- Made of smooth muscle, continuous with the inner circular muscle layer of the rectum.
- Involuntary control – contracts to maintain continence at rest.
- Located just beneath the mucosa, it forms a thickened ring of smooth muscle.

External Anal Sphincter (EAS)

- Composed of skeletal muscle, under voluntary control.
- Lies outside the IAS and is separated by intermuscular connective tissue (the intersphincteric space).

Common Location of Anal Fissures

- Posterior midline (6 o'clock position in lithotomy position) – most common site (~90%).
- Less frequently: anterior midline (12 o'clock), particularly in females.
- Rarely lateral, which might indicate secondary causes (e.g., Crohn's disease, malignancy, HIV).

Why posterior?

- Poorer blood supply to the posterior IAS makes it more vulnerable to ischemia and tearing.
- High resting pressure in the IAS increases shear forces during

defecation.

Clinical Relevance

- Fissures usually start in the anoderm, just distal to the dentate line.
- They extend longitudinally through the mucosa and may expose the underlying IAS fibers.
- Chronic fissures may show hypertrophied anal papillae, sentinel pile, and fibrotic IAS fibers.
- Laser tissue interaction chart showing depth vs. wavelength.
- Step by step intraoperative photos or line drawings of fiber positioning and energy delivery.
- Healing timeline diagram comparing laser vs. LIS phases.

Parikartika (Anal Fissure) – An Ayurvedic Surgical View

1. Nomenclature & Definition

- *Parikartika: "pari kṛta"* = torn or scraped by the passage of feces.
- Synonyms: *Chhedikā*, *Chedana* (tear), *Viṣkambha* (constriction).

2. Etiopathogenesis (Samprāpti)

2.1 Doṣa Involvement

सर्वे दोषा दुर्बलाहाराः.... व्यायामे.... मनोविकारैः प्रशामिते तथा ||

(Suśruta, Nidāna 11.15)

Imbalance of *Vāta* (mainly), *Pitta*, and *Kapha*, aggravated by:

- Ahaara viṣama (irregular diet)
- Divā swapna viṣama (sleep wake disturbance)
- Ati vyāyāma (over exercise)
- Ati brahmacarya (excessive sexual activity)
- Mano vikāra (stress, anger)

These lead to āma formation in the anorectal channel, drying of mucosa, and fissure formation under *Vata* driven spasm.

3. Lakṣaṇa (Clinical Features)

विभज्यमानं यदा तत्त्वङ्‌ लघुपरित्यागी....

(Charaka, Sūtra 20.28)

- Extreme, knife like pain at defecation (*Vāta* śola).
- Bleeding bright red drops on stool or paper (*Pitta* involvement).
- Spasmodic constriction of anus (*Vata* predominant).
- Sentinel pile (mucosal tag) and hypertrophied papilla (chronic).
- Constipation from fear of pain → vicious cycle.

4. Diagnosis (Parīkṣā)

- *Darśa* & *Sparśa*: Visual inspection under adequate light; palpation of sphincter tone.
- *Nadi Parīkṣā*: *Vāta-prakopa* pulse (irregular, rough).
- *Mutra Mala Netra Parīkṣā*: Evaluate systemic doṣa involvement (e.g., *Pitta* signs).

5. Management Overview

- *Saṃśodhana* (Purification): *Virechana* (purgation) if *Pitta* dominant.
- *Saṃśamana* (Pacification): *Snehana Swedana* (oil & fomentation), local *Kṣāra* application; *Basti* (medicated enema).
- *Śastra Karma* (Surgical Incision) for chronic, refractory cases.
- *ŚiroVirechana* in select *Pitta* aggravated fissures (to release heat).

6. *Śastra Karma* (Incisional Sphincterotomy)

6.1 Indications

- Chronic fissure > 6 weeks with fibrotic edges.

- Failure of *Kṣāra karma* and Sitz baths after 4–6 weeks.
- Marked sphincter hypertonia on palpation.

6.2 Instruments (Yantras & Śāstras)

Śastra (Cutting):

- *Śastraśāstra*: A fine, sharp anal knife (e.g., *Arśaparaṇa śastra*) with blade length 3–5 mm.
- *Mandalaśāstra*: Circular knife for precise, curved incision.

Yantra (Non cutting):

- *Karāṇḍī* (Probe): To gauge depth.
- *Kṣāraśodhaka yantra*: For chemical cauterization if needed.

Ancillary:

Gauze soaked in *Jatyādi Taila*, Blunt scissors, Sterile cotton swabs.

6.3 Dosage & Depth (Śastra Lakṣaṇa)

मांसलेषु३ यवमात्रं शस्त्रं निदध्यात....

(Suśruta, Śarīra 8.9)

- Insert blade to the depth of one yava (barley grain, ~2 mm) through inner sphincter fibers only.
- Length of incision: from the edge of fissure to submucosal tissue at sentinel pile.
- Direction: Posterior midline fissure → incision at 6 o'clock; anterior fissure → 12 o'clock.

6.4 Step by Step Technique

Anesthesia & Positioning

- Lithotomy or prone jackknife.
- Local infiltration: 2–3 mL of 0.5% bupivacaine around fissure edges.

Exposure

- Anoscope or proctoscope; gentle retraction of sentinel pile.

Incision

- Place blade tip at distal base of fissure.
- Advance 2 mm through hypertonic internal sphincter.
- Withdraw gradually, severing muscle fibers only (no mucosal excision).

Hemostasis

- Apply gauze with *Jatyādi Taila*; minimal bleeding expected.
- If oozing persists, sprinkle fine *Saindhava* (rock salt) or light *Kṣāra*.

Dress & Recover

- No sutures; allow mucosa to oppose naturally.
- Light gauze with *Taila*; advise patient to lie supine for 30 min

7. Kṣhāra Karma (Alkaline Debridement)

उच्छिद्य शोधनार्थं क्षारं दर्शयेत् उपचारिणः।

(Suśruta, Chikitsā Sthāna)

Apāmarga Kṣhāra paste applied to fissure bed for 1–2 minutes, then washed off.

Action: Chemical cauterization of fibrotic edges, reduction of muscle spasm, promotion of granulation.

8. Post Operative Care

8.1 Local Management

- Sitz Baths: 3 × daily with *Triphala* decoction (20 g *Triphala* in 1 L water).
- *Taila* Pichu: Gauze soaked in *Jatyādi Taila* or *Lajjalu Taila*, changed daily.

8.2 Internal Medications

Medicine	Formulation	Dose	Action
Aṣṭavarga Basti	Anuvasana Enema	60 mL, once daily for 7 days	*Vāta* pacification, healing
Nimbādi Guggulu	Tablet	500 mg, TID after meals	Anti inflammatory, anti edema
Śatavari + *Yashtimadhu*	Churna mix	5 g, BD with honey	Soothing, mucosal repair
Haridra (Turmeric)	*Churna*	1 g, TID with warm water	Anti inflammatory, anti microbial

8.3 Diet & Regimen

- Diet: Soft, easily digestible (*Yusha, Mudga kitchari*), high fiber (psyllium husk).
- Lifestyle: Avoid prolonged sitting; gentle walking; stress management.

9. *Rasāyana* & Long Term Prevention

- *Triphala Rasāyana*: 3 g at bedtime for 6 weeks—supports mucosal regeneration.
- *Guggulu*-based *Rasāyana*: *Yogarāja Guggulu* 250 mg, BD—for tissue repair and edema reduction.

Yoga & *Abhyānga*: Daily pelvic floor stretches; local *abhyānga* (oil massage) with *Mahanarayana Taila*.

10. Expected Outcomes & Complications

Parameter	Śastra Karma	Kṣāra Karma
Immediate pain relief	70–80% reduction	50–60% reduction
Healing time	2–3 weeks	3–4 weeks
Recurrence	< 5%	~ 10%
Fecal incontinence	< 1% (minor gas leak)	None
Local infection	< 2%	< 3%

1. Surgical Management of Anal Fistula (Bhagandara)

Modern Laser Surgery and Ayurvedic *Kṣhārasūtra* Integration

1. Introduction

Anal fistula is a chronic, abnormal epithelial tract connecting the anal canal or rectum to the perianal skin, often following an abscess. In Ayurveda, this is termed *Bhagandara*, listed among the *Ashtamahāgāda* (eight difficult-to-treat diseases).

अश्टौ महागदाः प्रोक्ता योपनास्ते चिकित्सकैः।

(Suśruta Saṃhitā, Sūtra Sthāna 33.4)

"*Bhagandara* is one of the eight major diseases considered *krichchhra-sādhya* (difficult to cure)."

2. Etiopathogenesis

Modern View:

- Originates from infected anal glands (cryptoglandular theory).
- Leads to abscess formation → ruptures → fistulous tract.
- Tracts may be simple or complex, involving sphincter muscles.

Ayurvedic View:

भगे निपीड्य मांसं यद् भिद्यते नाडिवद् बहिः। स्याच्छोणितं पुरिषं वा स भगेन्दरो निगद्यते।।

(Aṣṭāṅga Hṛdaya, Nidāna Sthāna 10.6)

"When the tissue between the anus and perineum breaks and discharges blood or feces like a tubular tract, it is called Bhagandara."

3. Classification

Modern Classification (Parks):

1. Core Classifications

1.1 Parks (Surgical/Anatomic) Classification – "What you cut is what you get"

Type	Anatomy	% of fistulae	Sphincter involvement	Key Surgical Considerations	Typical Op
Inters-phincteric	Track in intersphincteric plane; internal opening at dentate line, external opening perianal	~55%	None (external sphincter preserved)	Low risk to continence; fistulotomy usually curative	Lay-open (fistulotomy)
Transs-phincteric	Track passes through external sphincter into ischiorectal fossa then to skin	~30%	Partial EAS division	Risk ↑ with high trans-sphincteric (>30–50 % EAS)	Low: fistulotomy; High: seton, LIFT, advancement flap
Supras-phincteric	Track ascends in intersphincteric plane, crosses over puborectalis, descends through levator into ischiorectal fossa	5–10%	Entire EAS but not IAS	Fistulotomy contra-indicated; need sphincter-sparing	LIFT, seton + staged, advancement flap, VAAFT
Extras-phincteric	Track originates in rectum/ sigmoid, traverses levator and ischiorectal fat to skin; sphincters not pierced	<1% (rare)	Nil (passes outside complex)	Usually secondary to trauma, Crohn's, foreign body; mandate proximal source control	Resection of tract ± flap; treat underlying pathology

Note: "High" fistula = crosses >30–50 % of external sphincter or above dentate line; carries higher incontinence risk.

1.2 MRI / St-James's University Hospital Classification (Radiologist-friendly)

Grades 1–5 correspond closely to Parks but add abscess/sepsis detail:

1 = Simple intersphincteric; 2 = Intersphincteric with abscess/ secondary track; 3 = Transsphincteric; 4 = Transsphincteric with abscess; 5 = Suprasphincteric / Extrasphincteric. MRI is ≥90 % sensitive for mapping, now standard pre-op in complex cases (NICE 2022).

1.3 Etiologic / Disease-based

- Cryptoglandular (≈90 %)
- Crohn's-related (10–15 %) – often multiple, high, active proctitis → medical ± surgical
- Obstetric, radiation, trauma, malignancy, tuberculosis, hidradenitis suppurativa

2. Diagnostic Work-up & Criteria

1. History: recurrent abscess, purulent drainage, pain.
2. Inspection & digital rectal exam – note external opening, cord-like tract, goodsall's rule.
3. Anoscopy/proctoscopy to identify internal opening.
4. Imaging if complex, recurrent, anterior in female, Crohn's, prior surgery, or incontinence risk:
    - Pelvic MRI with endoanal coil (Gold standard)
    - Endoanal ultrasound (good for simple fistulae)
    - CT fistulography if MRI unavailable
5. Labs: CRP, Hb, albumin (Crohn's), HbA1c (diabetics) – affects healing.

3. Red Flags & Complications

- Recurrent perianal sepsis/abscess
- Fecal incontinence risk (high tracts, women, multiparity)
- Associated Crohn's proctitis – worsens outcome
- Malignant transformation (rare; suspect if chronic non-healing >5 y)

- Extrasphincteric track – search for colorectal malignancy or foreign body

4. Management Overview (Evidence-Based 2024)

- Acute abscess: prompt incision & drainage ± seton placement if tract obvious (ACPGBI 2023).
- Definitive fistula surgery after sepsis resolution and mapping. Choice depends on Parks type, height, continence status:

Strategy	Indication	Success	Continence Impact
Fistulotomy/lay-open	Low inter-/trans-sphincteric (<1/3 EAS)	90–95 %	Minimal
Cutting seton (rare use now)	High trans-	80 %	Up to 35 % incontinence
Loose seton (silk/silastic)	Sepsis control, Crohn's, staged	N/A (bridging)	Low
LIFT (ligation of intersphincteric track)	High trans- & supra-	70–80 %	Low (<10 %)
Mucosal/advancement flap	High tracts, Crohn's	60–80 %	<10 %
VAAFT (video-assisted anal fistula tx)	Complex, recurrent	70 %	Minimal
FiLaC®/laser closure	Selected centers	60–80 %	Minimal
Plugs (bioprosthetic) / fibrin glue	Crohn's, sphincter preservation	30–50 %	None
Autologous or allogenic MSC (darvadstrocel 2019 ADMIRE trial)	Crohn's complex fistula	56 % closure at 52 wks	None

Crohn's disease: combine biologics (anti-TNF, ustekinumab, vedolizumab) with seton (AGA 2022 strong recommendation).

Post-op care: stool softener, sitz baths, avoid opioids, early follow-up.

5. Surveillance & Follow-up

- Review 2 weeks to assess wound, drainage.
- MRI at 3–6 m in complex cases to document healing.
- Continence assessment (Wexner score) pre- and post-op.
- If persistent sepsis, consider re-imaging and staged revision.

6. Differential Diagnoses to Keep in Mind

- Hidradenitis suppurativa sinus
- Anal fissure with sentinel abscess
- Pilonidal sinus extending cranially
- Bartholin duct cyst/fistula (in females)
- Malignancy (anal adenocarcinoma or squamous) – biopsy chronic tracts

Types of fistula in ano by Ayurveda (Suhruta):

Ayurvedic texts (mainly *Sushruta Samhita* and *Charaka Samhita*) describe the same entity as "*Bhagandara*" and stratify it by *Dosha* predominance and macroscopic pattern of the tract's external opening(s).

Given you are likely reviewing complementary frameworks (e.g., for patients who request traditional insights or when considering *Kṣārasūtra* therapy), below is a concise, clinically oriented summary.

Ayurvedic classification of Bhagandara

System	Sub-types	Canonical description (Sushruta/ Charaka)	Practical correlates
1. *Doṣaja* (humoral) types	• *Vātaja* • *Pittaja* • *Kaphaja* • *Sannipātaja (tri-Dosha)* • *Kṣataja* (traumatic/post-injury)	Defined by dominant *Dosha* symptoms—pain & dryness (V), burning & bleeding (P), induration & mucous discharge (K); Sannipātaja is mixed/severe; Kṣataja follows injury/iatrogenic cause	Correspond to inflammatory tone, discharge character. No anatomic basis, but sometimes quoted to guide choice of medications, Sitz baths (Avagāha-sveda) and topical lepa
2. *Mārga-bheda* (tract pattern) types (Sushruta's "*pañca-vidha*")	1. *Śataponaka* ("100 openings") 2. *Pāriśrāvi* ("profuse dribbling") 3. *Śaṃbhūka-varta* ("conch-shaped/spiral") 4. *Unmārga* ("false/ectopic tract") 5. *Ṛju bhagandara* ("straight tract")	Multiplicity of external openings, continuous thin serous discharge, cork-screw tract, opening into urethra/vagina/ rectum, and single straight low tract respectively	Closest to modern concepts of complex branching fistula, high fistula with persistent discharge, horseshoe or spiral high supra-, extrasphincteric, and simple low inter-/submucosal respectively
3. Complication-based variants (later texts)	"*Udar-bhagandara*" (extending into abdomen), "*Guda-bhagandara*" (perianal), etc.	Reflect extension beyond anorectal ring	Rarely cited today

Key point: these typologies pre-date sphincteric anatomy knowledge; their practical utility lies mainly in "*Kṣārasūtra*" (medicated seton) therapy selection, prognostication, and *Dosha*-tailored adjuvants (e.g., *Triphalā-Guggulu*, *Jatyādi Taila*).

Modern evidence for Ayurvedic interventions

- *Kṣārasūtra* vs fistulotomy
  - Meta-analysis of 6 RCTs (n≈410) showed comparable long-term healing (≈85 %) but longer time-to-closure (6-8 wk) with *Kṣārasūtra*; however, lower incontinence risk (0–2 %) versus conventional fistulotomy (4–10 %). (Int J Colorectal Dis 2022)
  - Most data are low-to-moderate quality; heterogeneity in tract complexity.

- Adjunct herbal formulations: Minimal controlled data; predominantly case series.

Current guidelines (ASCRS 2023) recognise *Kṣārasūtra* as an option in resource-limited settings for low, simple tracts provided the surgeon is trained and the patient counseled re: prolonged dressing changes.

Red-flags & when Ayurveda alone is unsafe

1. High trans-/suprasphincteric or extrasphincteric tracts
2. Associated Crohn's disease, TB, malignancy
3. Acute sepsis/abscess, immunocompromise
4. Fecal incontinence risk factors or prior sphincter surgery

Such cases warrant MRI pelvis, multidisciplinary input and advanced surgical options (LIFT, VAAFT, advancement flap, seton with staged sphincter division).

Integrated management algorithm

1. Confirm anatomy: MRI or endo-US → Parks classification.
2. If low/simple: choose fistulotomy, LIFT, or *Kṣārasūtra* (with informed consent re healing time).
3. If complex/high: staging with draining seton ± biologics (if Crohn), followed by sphincter-saving procedure.
4. Monitor healing (weekly) and ensure glycaemic control, smoking cessation, Sitz baths.
5. Re-image if persistent discharge >12 wk or new tract openings (*Śataponaka* phenotype).

4. Modern Laser Surgery (Filac – Fistula Laser Closure)

- Principle:

Using 1470 nm radial diode laser, energy is delivered circumferentially, destroying the epithelium and sealing the tract.

- *Equipment:*
  - Radial fiber laser probe
  - Diode laser unit (10–15 watts)
  - Seton (if required), irrigation cannula, endoscopic fistula probe

- *Step-by-Step Laser Procedure:*
  - Diagnosis: Clinical exam, MRI or Endoanal Ultrasound.
  - Anesthesia: Regional or General
  - Internal opening identification: Probing and irrigation
  - Laser Probe Insertion: Through external opening, up to internal

  - Laser Application:
    - Power: 10–12 Watts (continuous wave)
    - Withdrawal Rate: 1 mm/sec

  - Closure: Internal opening sealed or left to granulate

- *Advantages:*

Feature	Laser Surgery (FiLaC)
Minimally invasive	✓ Yes
Sphincter safety	✓ Preserved
Healing time	✓ Fast (2–3 weeks)
Pain	✓ Minimal
Recurrence	✗ Lower (10–20%)
Hospital stay	✓ Day-care possible

Perianal fistula surgery has shifted toward sphincter-preserving techniques. Among these, the Fistula-tract Laser Closure (FiLaC®) and related laser ablation methods (LAFT, OTSC-Laser) use a radial-emitting diode laser fiber to coagulate and collapse the tract from the internal opening outward, aiming for durable closure while avoiding continence impairment.

1. Patient Selection & Pre-operative Work-up

Step	**Key Points**	**Evidence/ Guideline**
Classification	Parks or St. James MRI grading; FiLaC best suited for inter-/trans-sphincteric tracts ≤3–4 cm; horseshoe tracts may need staged approach	ESCP 2023
Imaging	Endo-anal US ± hydrogen peroxide or MRI pelvis to map all tracts/abscesses	Strong recommendation
Sepsis Control	Drain acute abscess; consider loose seton 4–6 w if high trans-sphincteric or Crohn's	CRICS 2022
Contra-indications	Malignancy in tract, active proctitis, >50 % sphincter circumference lost, anorectal strictures	–

2. Equipment & Laser Parameters

Item	Typical Spec	Notes
Laser generator	Diode 1470 nm (some use 980 nm)	Water absorption peak → confined thermal spread (~2–3 mm)
Fiber	360° radial emitting, 400–600 μm core	Sterile, single-use
Power	10–15 W continuous	Adjust for tract diameter
Pull-back rate	1 mm / s (≈1 cm in 10 s)	Use metronome/foot pedal pulses
Ancillary	Dilators, fistula probe, irrigation cannula, diathermy or stapler for internal opening closure (optional)	

3. Operative Technique (FiLaC®) – Step-by-Step

1. Position: Lithotomy or prone jack-knife; prophylactic antibiotics (2nd-gen ceph ± MTZ).
2. Internal opening identification: via gentle probe or methylene blue/H_2O_2 instillation.
3. Curettage/brush: Light mechanical debridement; avoid excessive wall trauma.
4. Flush & dry: Saline irrigation then compressed air to keep tract patent.
5. Laser fiber insertion: Introduce to abscess cavity or external opening end.
6. Energy delivery: Activate laser while slow, steady pull-back to internal opening (≈8–12 s/cm).
7. Closure of internal opening (optional but ↑success)
    - 3-0 Vicryl Z-stitch, anoderm flap, or OTSC clip.

8. External opening management: Leave open for drainage or loosely closed with interrupted absorbables.
9. Dressings: Non-occlusive; no packing needed.

Mean operative time: 15–25 min.

4. Post-operative Care & Monitoring

Day/ Week	Task	Rationale
POD 0–1	Same-day discharge common; analgesia with NSAID ± acetaminophen	Minimal pain expected
1 w	Review wound, rule-out abscess	Early sepsis detection
6 w	Clinical exam ± EUA if symptoms	Primary healing check
3 mo	MRI or EAUS if doubts	Detect occult persistence
≥6 mo	Assess continence (Wexner score) & QoL	Document sphincter safety

Advise Sitz baths, fiber 25–30 g/day, avoid strenuous exertion 2 w.

5. Outcomes & Evidence

Study / Meta-analysis	n	Primary Healing	Continence Impact	Notes
Wilhelm 2011 (orig.)	11	81 % @24 mo	None	Pilot
Emile et al. 2022 SR (24 studies)	1,835	67 % pooled (range 40–94 %)	0.8 % new incontinence	Higher success if internal opening closed

D'Hoore RCT 2023 (FiLaC vs LIFT)	97	73 % vs 76 % @12 mo (ns)	Continence unchanged in both	FiLaC shorter LOS
NICE IPG 650 2019	–	Evidence adequate for short-term efficacy; recommend audit	Call for registry data	

Predictors of failure: Crohn's disease, horseshoe, multiple secondary tracts, no internal closure, prior radiation.

6. Complications & Pitfalls

- Early abscess (<5 %) → treat with drainage ± antibiotics
- Bleeding/hematoma (<1 %)
- Temporary flare of discharge (first 2 wk) – usually inflammatory debris
- Skin burn if fiber not within tract – keep tactile feedback constant
- Recurrence median 4–6 mo; consider repeat FiLaC or alternative (VAAFT, LIFT, advancement flap)

7. How It Compares Clinically

Metric	**FiLaC**	**Fistulotomy**	**LIFT**	**VAAFT**
Continence risk	<1 %	10–40 % (high tracts)	0–5 %	<2 %
Healing (%)	60–80	90–95 (low tract)	70–80	70–80
Re-do friendly	Yes	Limited	Yes	Yes
Technical learning	Moderate	Low	Moderate	High

Use FiLaC primarily for high trans-sphincteric or complex *fistulas* where fistulotomy is hazardous.

DLPEL ("Distal Laser + Proximal Ligation") -

Complex (high trans-sphincteric, supra- or extra-sphincteric, recurrent, horseshoe) fistula-in-ano poses two competing goals: 1) durable sepsis eradication and 2) preservation of continence. "Distal Laser + Proximal Ligation" (DLPL; occasionally written DLPeL/DLPEL) is a hybrid sphincter-saving technique that combines a FiLaC-style diode-laser ablation of the distal tract with ligation of the tract at the inter-sphincteric plane. It seeks to harness the predictable closure rates of LIFT while adding the tract-obliterating benefits of laser energy, particularly in long or ramifying fistulae.

Anatomical & Diagnostic Snapshot

- Classify with MRI or 3-D EAUS (gold standard for extensions ± abscess).
- High trans-sphincteric, supra-sphincteric, recurrent tracts are the prime DLPL candidates.
- Exclude Crohn-related, malignancy-associated, TB, or radiation fistulae; outcome data for these groups are sparse.

DLPL – Operative Protocol (Evidence-based Outline)

Step	Key Technical Points	Pearls / Pitfalls
1. Pre-op Sepsis Control	Loose draining seton 4-6 w if acute abscess or heavy discharge.	Reduces post-laser abscess risk.
2. Anaesthesia & Position	RA/GA; lithotomy; prophylactic antibiotics (single-dose 2nd-gen ceph ± metronidazole).	Maintain normothermia.
3. Internal Opening (IO) Identification	Probing + hydrogen peroxide/ methylene blue; confirm on MRI images.	If IO elusive, abandon DLPL.
4. Proximal Ligation (inter-sphincteric plane)	Circumferential dissection of tract at IO via small inter-sphincteric incision; ligate with 2-0 polyglactin; divide tract distal to ligature.	Secure tie without injuring IAS/EAS.

5. Distal Laser Ablation	Introduce 1470 nm radial-emitting fibre through external opening; 10 W, pull-back 1 cm/3 s, until ligated stump.	Maintain tract patency (no curette) to allow uniform energy delivery.
6. External Opening	Left open ± small wick; no primary closure.	Facilitates drainage → ↓abscess.
7. Post-op Care	Day-care/overnight; NSAIDs; sitz baths; soft diet; stool-softener x 1 wk.	Resume desk work in 2–3 d.

Outcomes & Evidence

Study / Series	n	Fistula Type	Healing @12–18 mo	Re-op Rate	Incontinence
Garg P. et al, Int J Colorectal Dis 2021	70	Complex	88 %	4 %	0 %
Garg P. multi-centre, Dis Colon Rectum 2022	200	Mixed	90 %	6 %	0 %
Systematic Review, Colorectal Dis 2023	6 studies, 412 pts	Complex & recurrent	Pooled 86 % (CI 78–92)	7 %	<1 % transient soiling

Level of evidence: IIb (prospective cohorts); RCTs awaited.

Comparators (approximate healing rates):

- LIFT 70-80 %; FiLaC 60-70 %; VAAFT 65-75 %; Advancement flap 60-80 %; traditional seton 50-70 % with variable incontinence.

Patient Selection – Practical Checklist

1. Complex cryptoglandular fistula with single identifiable IO.
2. No active Crohn's, TB, neoplasm, or uncontrolled sepsis.
3. BMI < 35 and good sphincter tone (manometry optional).
4. Patient accepts need for MRI follow-up and possibility of second procedure if recurrence.

Peri-operative Red Flags / Complications

- Failure to find/ligate IO – switch to staged seton or classic LIFT.
- Early post-op abscess (≈3–5 %) – prompt drainage, consider re-seton.
- Recurrence usually at IO; evaluate with MRI; second DLPL/ LIFT feasible.
- Incontinence is rare (<1 %) – still counsel thoroughly, especially if prior fistulotomies.

Follow-up Algorithm

- 1 wk: wound check, pain control, bowel regimen
- 6 wk: clinical healing, discontinue sitz if dry
- 3 mo: MRI if symptoms or complex anatomy
- 6 & 12 mo: symptom-directed visit; DRE ± EAUS
- Beyond 12 mo: discharge to GP with instructions to return for any new discharge or pain.

Filac Animation

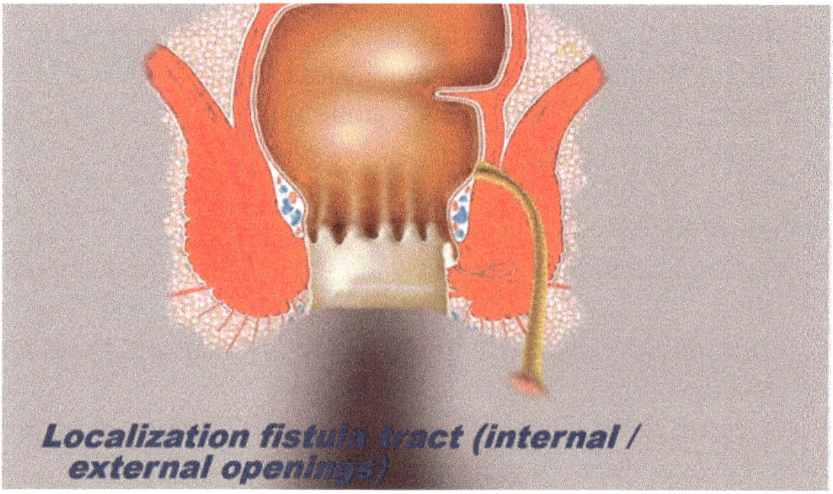

Laser Fiber Insertion

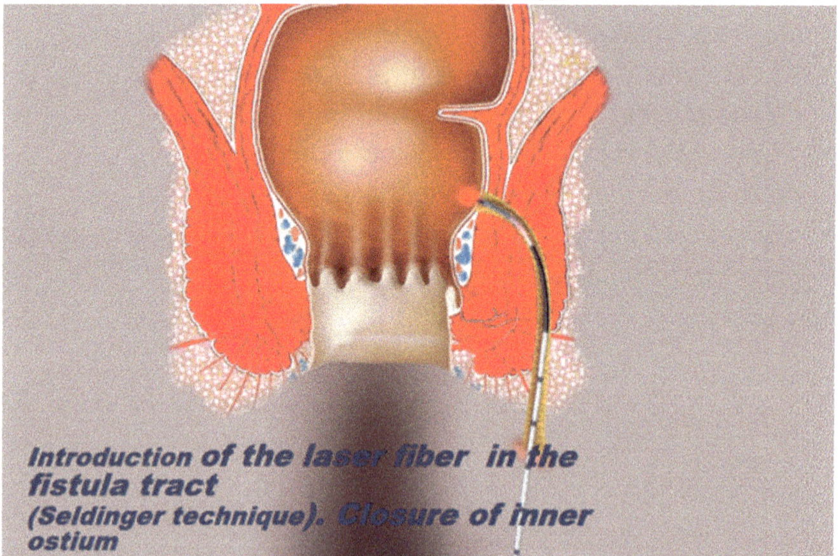

Laser Ablation In 360 Degree

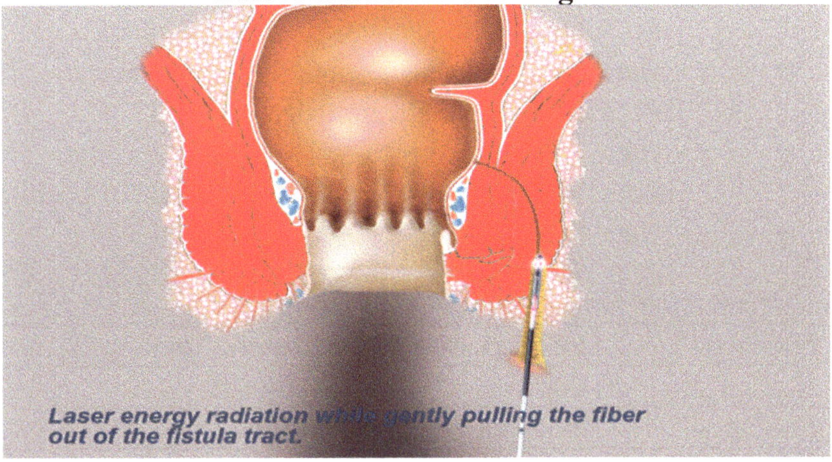

5. AYURVEDA MANAGEMENT – *Kshārasūtra* Therapy

- ***Classical Text:***

भगन्दरं च कर्षन्ति सूत्रेण क्षारपङ्कजम्।

(Suśruta Chikitsā Sthāna 17.31)

"The tract of *Bhagandara* is managed with a *Kṣārasūtra* which cuts and heals simultaneously."

- ***Materials***:
  - *Apāmarga Kṣāra* (alkaline ash)
  - *Snuhi Kṣīra* (latex)
  - *Haridra Chūrṇa* (turmeric powder)

- ***Mechanism*:**

छेद्यं भेद्यं लेख्यं च शोधनं रोपणं तथा।

(Suśruta Chikitsā Sthāna 17.29)

"*Kṣārasūtra* acts as cutting, draining, scraping, disinfecting, and healing agent."

- ***Procedure:***
  - Tract Probing with a malleable metallic probe.
  - *Kṣhārasūtra* Insertion through the fistula tract.
  - Thread Tie: Loop tied externally.
  - Weekly Changes: Thread replaced every 5–7 days.
  - Gradual Cutting: Tract is cut over 4–6 weeks, healing by secondary intention.

6. Comparative Table – LASER vs Ksharasutra

Parameter	**FiLaC (Laser)**	**Ksharasutra Therapy**
Hospital Stay	Day care	OPD/Day care
Healing Time	2–3 weeks	4–6 weeks
Pain	Minimal	Moderate (esp. during thread change)
Recurrence Rate	~15–20%	~10–15%
Continence Risk	Very Low	Low to moderate (in complex tracts)
Accessibility	Expensive equipment	Affordable & available

7. Integrative Approach (Laser + Ayurveda)

Phase	**Modern Intervention**	**Ayurvedic Support**
Pre-op	MRI, antibiotics	*Deepana (Trikatu), Pāchana (Triphala)*
Surgery	FiLaC procedure	*Kṣāra lepa or Taila post-op*
Post-op	Analgesics, Sitz bath	*Jatyādi Taila, Triphalā kwātha*
Rasāyana	Nutritional support	*Haridra, Guggulu, Ashwagandhā*

8. Post-Operative Ayurvedic Care

- ***Internal Medications:***
  - *Guggulu*–Tikta Ghṛta – Anti-inflammatory
  - *Haridra Chūrṇa* – 1 g with warm water TID
  - *Triphala Chūrṇa* – 3 g at night for gut detox
  - Ashwagandhā *Rasāyana* – For tissue recovery

- ***Local Care:***
    - *Triphala* Sitz bath – Twice daily
    - *Jatyādi Taila* pichu – Applied over healing tract
    - *Manjishṭhādi Lepa* – If induration exists

9. KEY SANSKRIT SHLOKAS (with translation)

- ***Definition:***

भगे निपीड्य मांसं यद् भिद्यते नाडिवद् बहिः।

(Aṣṭāṅga Hṛdaya, Nidāna Sthāna 10.6)

"Fistulous tract emerging around anus and genitals is Bhagandara."

- ***Kṣhārasūtra Benefits:***

छेद्यं भेद्यं लेख्यं च शोधनं रोपणं तथा।

(Suśruta Chikitsā 17.29)

"Kṣāra performs incision, drainage, scraping, purification, and healing."

- ***Importance of Kṣhārasūtra:***

भगन्दरं च कर्षन्ति सूत्रेण क्षारपङ्कजम्।

(Suśruta Chikitsā 17.31)

"Bhagandara is to be treated by alkaline medicated thread."

Anal *Fistula* Management Landscape

Most clinicians now stratify fistula-in-ano by the Parks/St. James MRI classifications and choose either a lay-open procedure (fistulotomy) for simple, low tracts or a sphincter-preserving technique (LIFT, seton, VAAFT, FiLaC, advancement flap, OTSC, etc.) for complex/high tracts to avoid incontinence.

Within the Ayurvedic/para-surgical armamentarium, *Kṣārasūtra* (medicated seton) therapy has a long history in India. "IFTAK" (Interception of Fistulous Tract with Application of *Kṣārasūtra*) is a modified, minimally invasive variant aimed at reducing pain, healing time, and sphincter injury compared with the classical technique.

Where IFTAK Fits

- Concept: Instead of threading the entire primary tract, a small "interception window" is created near the external opening; only the segment from that window to the internal opening is threaded with *Kṣārasūtra*.
- Ideal anatomy: Simple or low-lying trans-/intersphincteric tracts with a single internal opening located within 2 cm of the dentate line.
- Relative contraindications: Suprasphincteric/extrasphincteric, horseshoe, multiple secondary extensions, Crohn-related, active abscess, sphincter fibrosis.

Pre-operative Work-up

5. Mapping – Gentle probe, hydrogen peroxide–methylene blue injection, and preferably an MRI pelvis (St James grading) if >1 tract or prior surgery.
6. Screen for Crohn's, TB, diabetes.
7. Routine labs, HIV/HBsAg/HCV where relevant.
8. Bowel prep: single dose PEG or phosphate enema the evening prior; clear-liquid breakfast day of surgery.

Step-by-Step Technique (IFTAK)

Step	Key Technical Points & Pearls
1. Anaesthesia	Saddle/caudal block or short GA; lithotomy or prone jack-knife.
2. Identification	Dilate anal canal gently; identify internal opening with proctoscope. If not visible, inject dilute methylene blue through external opening.
3. Interception window	Make a 1.5–2 cm curvilinear incision over the primary tract ~1 cm lateral to the anal verge (usually 1–1.5 cm proximal to the external opening).
4. Tract deroofing (distal segment)	Excise/deroof the distal 1–2 cm tract segment to allow dependent drainage—this part heals by secondary intention.
5. Threading proximal tract	Pass a malleable probe from the internal opening out through the interception window. Tie the *kṣārasūtra* (barbour linen no. 20 coated with *snuhi kṣīra* + *apāmārgakṣāra*) in situ, forming a loop only across the proximal tract.
6. Haemostasis & closure	No sphincter muscle is divided; minimal cautery. Leave interception window open; pack lightly with 5% povidone-iodine gauze.
7. Post-op seton change	Weekly change/rail-roading of fresh *kṣārasūtra* until the loop cuts through (~0.5 cm/week) and tract heals (median 4-6 weeks).

Post-operative Care & Monitoring

- Sitz baths (warm water + povidone) 10 min TID
- NSAIDs or *tramadol* as needed; avoid opioids >48 h
- High-fibre diet, stool-softeners for 2 weeks
- Weekly OPD review: inspect for granulation, discharge, and change the *Kṣārasūtra*

- Red flags: fever, increasing pain/swelling (exclude abscess), early widening of defect (incontinence risk)

Outcomes & Evidence

Study / Series	n	Primary Healing	Recurrence	Incontinence
Dwivedi et al, AYU 2013	45	93% at 8 wk	4%	0%
Nanal et al, J Ayurveda 2016	38 (RCT vs conventional *kṣārasūtra*)	89% vs 82%	5% vs 11%	0%
Upadhyay et al, IJAS 2020	60	95%	3%	0%

Evidence quality: predominantly single-center, non-blinded case series; no large multicentre RCTs. Level III evidence; strong need for high-quality comparative trials versus LIFT/VAAFT.

Reported advantages

- Mean pain score POD1: 3–4/10 vs 6–7/10 (conventional)
- Mean total cutting/healing time: 4–6 weeks vs 8–12 weeks
- Better patient comfort—no external thread across perianal skin

Limitations

- Limited evidence outside Ayurveda centers
- Operator dependent; unfamiliar to colorectal surgeons trained in Western techniques
- Unclear long-term (>5 y) recurrence data

Comparison With Other Sphincter-Preserving Techniques

Parameter	IFTAK	LIFT	VAAFT	FiLaC
Tech base	*Kṣārasūtra* (chemical seton)	Surgical ligation	Endoscopic	Laser energy
Healing time	4–6 wk	6–8 wk	6–10 wk	4–6 wk
Reported continence impairment	Rare (0-1%)	0-2%	0-2%	0-1%
Recurrence (literature range)	3-10%	6-15%	5-20%	6-15%
Cost & instrumentation	Very low	Low-mod	High	High
Evidence grade	III	II	II	II

Pitfalls & Complications

- Missed secondary tract
  1. recurrence

- Chemical burn if *Kṣārasūtra* contacts perianal skin; protect with zinc oxide

- Tight thread
  1. early cut-through
  2. sphincter injury

- Inadequate weekly change
  1. ineffective chemical action, persistent tract
- Patient non-adherence to follow-up

Patient Education Pearls (lay language)

"Your fistula is a small tunnel between your bowel and skin.

We will remove the infected end near the skin and place a

medicated thread only in the deeper portion. The thread slowly cuts and heals the tunnel from inside over 4–6 weeks. You will come once a week for dressing and thread change. Keep the area clean with warm baths, eat high-fibre foods to avoid strain, and call us if you develop fever, severe pain, or new swelling."

Key References

1. Dwivedi V et al. AYU (2013);34:143-7.
2. Nanal S et al. J Ayurveda Integr Med (2016);7:7-12 (RCT).
3. Upadhyay S et al. Indian J Ayur Surg (2020);1:45-51.
4. Ommer A. "Sphincter-preserving techniques for high anal fistula." Colorectal Dis 2021.
5. IAPSCON Guidelines on *Kṣārasūtra* Therapy, 2022 edition

10. CONCLUSION

The modern laser technique (FiLaC) offers a sphincter-preserving, fast-recovery option with minimal pain, while *Kṣārasūtra* therapy is a time-tested Ayurvedic method with proven efficacy and low recurrence.

Combining both approaches, under expert guidance, ensures holistic care, faster recovery, lower recurrence, and better patient satisfaction.

Certainly. Below is a fully detailed, structured, and clinically comprehensive explanation of Anal Fistula (*Bhagandara*) surgical management, integrating:

- Modern proctology (with a focus on Laser/Fistula Laser Closure - FiLaC),
- Ayurvedic surgery (particularly *Kṣhārasūtra* therapy), and
- Classical Sanskrit ślokas from Suśruta, Caraka, and *Aṣṭāṅga Hṛdaya.*
- Anal Fistula (*Bhagandara*): Integrative Surgical Approach – Modern Laser & Ayurveda

1. **Section 1: What Is An Anal Fistula?**

- ***Modern Medical Definition:***

An anal fistula is an abnormal tract or tunnel that forms between the anal canal and the perianal skin due to chronic infection of anal glands.

    - Typically follows an anorectal abscess.
    - Symptoms: pus or stool discharge, pain, swelling, recurrent infections.

- ***Ayurvedic Description – Bhagandara:***

भगे निपीड्य मांसं यद् भिद्यते नाडिवद् बहिः।
स्याच्छोणितं पुरिषं वा स भगेन्दरो निगद्यते।।

(Aṣṭāṅga Hṛdaya, Nidāna 10.6)

"When the flesh near the anus bursts open like a sinus and discharges blood or feces, it is called *Bhagandara*."

2. **Section 2: Classifications**

- ***Modern (Parks Classification):***

Type	Description
Intersphincteric	Tract lies between internal & external sphincter
Transsphincteric	Crosses both sphincters
Suprasphincteric	Extends above the external sphincter
Extrasphincteric	Outside the sphincter complex

- Types of *Bhagandara* by Ayurveda :

वातपित्तकफैश्चैव त्रिभिर्दोषैरसम्भवैः।
सन्निपातेन जातोऽयं स भगेन्दरो महागदः।।

(Suśhruta, Nidāna 4.5)

Type	Predominant Doṣa	Clinical Features
Vātaja	*Vāta*	Dry tract, intense pain, narrow
Pittaja	*Pitta*	Burning, redness, pus discharge
Kaphaja	*Kapha*	Sticky discharge, itching
Sannipātaja	*Tri-doṣa*	Mixed symptoms, chronic, difficult
Śārīrabhavaja	*Congenital*	Present from birth (rectovaginal, etc.)

3. Section 3: Modern Surgical Management

- ***FiLaC (Fistula Laser Closure)***

A minimally invasive, sphincter-preserving technique using a 1470 nm radial laser probe.

Step-by-Step Procedure:

- Evaluation: MRI/endoanal ultrasound to assess tract.
  - Anesthesia: Spinal or general.
  - Probing: Tract identified and cleaned.
  - Laser Fiber Insertion: Radial fiber introduced from external to internal opening.

- Laser Activation:
  - Power: 10–12 watts
  - Withdrawal rate: ~1 mm/sec

Closure of Internal Opening: Optionally closed with sutures or flap.

Benefits:

- No cutting or excision
- Low risk of incontinence
- Fast recovery (3–7 days)
- Cosmetically clean
- Low recurrence (~15%)

4. Section 4: Ayurvedic Surgical Management

Kshārasūtra Therapy – The Ayurvedic Gold Standard

क्षारसूत्रेण भगन्दरं
कर्षयित्वा विशुद्धिम् आप्नोति ।।

(Suśruta Chikitsā 17.31)

"By passing a *Kṣārasūtra* through the tract, the *Bhagandara* is purified and cured."

Contents of Kshārasūtra:

- *Apāmarga Kṣāra* – caustic alkaline agent
- Snuhi Kṣīra – latex from Euphorbia nerifolia
- *Haridra* (Turmeric) – antimicrobial and healing

Procedure:

- Tract is probed using a malleable instrument.
- A medicated thread (*Kṣārasūtra*) is passed through.
- Thread is tightened weekly – slowly cuts, cauterizes, and heals.
- Entire tract is destroyed and replaced by healthy tissue.

छेद्यं भेद्यं लेख्यं च शोधनं रोपणं तथा।
येन स्यान्निःस्पृहो रोगो क्षारः स परिकीर्तितः ।।

(Suśhruta, Chikitsā 17.29)

"That which cuts, scrapes, cleanses, and heals – is the true *Kshāra (alkali)*."

5. Section 5: Comparison – Modern Laser Vs Ksharasūtra

Feature	**FiLaC Laser**	***Kṣhārasūtra* Therapy**
Invasiveness	Minimal (Non-excisional)	Minimal (Thread-based)
Healing Time	2–3 weeks	4–6 weeks
Sphincter Damage	None	Slight risk in deep tracts

Pain Post-op	Mild	Moderate (during weekly changes)
Recurrence Rate	10–15%	5–10%
Cost	High (equipment)	Low (herbal materials)
Procedure Complexity	Requires expertise	Easy in Ayurvedic OPD settings

6. Section 6: Integrative Post-Operative Management

Internal Ayurvedic Medications:

Medicine	Purpose
Triphala Churna	Gut detox, regular bowel habits
Haridra	Anti-inflammatory, wound healing
Guggulu	Anti-microbial, deep tissue healing
Ashwagandhā	Nervine support, stress modulation

- Local Applications:
  - *Jatyādi Taila* / Seetodaka *Taila* – for wound healing
  - *Triphala Kwātha* Sitz bath – antiseptic and soothing
  - Lepa of *Manjishṭhā* and *Nimba* – reduces local swelling

7. Section 7: Key Sanskrit *Shlokas*

Topic	***Śhloka (*Transliterated*)***	Source
Definition of *Bhagandara*	***Bhage nipīḍya māṁsaṁ yad bhidyate nāḍivad bahiḥ…***	*Aṣṭāṅga Hṛdaya, Nidāna 10.6*
Kṣhārasūtra Therapy	***Bhagandaraṁ ca karṣanti sūtreṇa*** *kṣārapaṅkajāḥ*…	*Suśruta Chikitsā 17.31*
Five Actions of *Kṣhāra*	*Chhedyaṁ* ***bhedyaṁ lekhyaṁ ca*** *śodhanaṁ* ***ropaṇaṁ tathā…***	*Suśruta Chikitsā 17.29*
Mahāgāda (Incurables)	***Aṣṭau mahāgadāḥ proktāḥ yopanaste cikitsakaiḥ – Arśaḥ, Bhagandaraḥ…***	*Suśruta Sūtra 33.4*

8. Section 8: Conclusion

Both modern laser FiLaC and Ayurvedic *Kṣārasūtra* offer effective, sphincter-safe treatments for anal fistula (*Bhagandara*).

An integrated approach that uses laser for clean tract closure and Ayurvedic medicines for post-op detox, healing, and recurrence prevention ensures:

- Faster recovery
- Less recurrence
- Holistic healing

Clinical Case Studies:

Here are two real-style clinical case studies of Anal Fistula (*Bhagandara*) treatment—one using Modern Laser Surgery (FiLaC) and the other using Ayurvedic *Kṣārasūtra* therapy. These can be used in your book chapter, research publication, or presentation to illustrate integrative clinical success.

Clinical Case Study 1: Laser Surgery (FiLaC) in High Transsphincteric Anal Fistula

Patient Profile:

- Name: Mr. Rahul S.
- Age/Gender: 38 years, Male
- Occupation: IT Professional
- Presenting Complaint: Recurrent pus discharge near anal region for 6 months, occasional fever and pain.

Diagnosis:

- Type: High Transsphincteric Fistula
- Investigations:
    - MRI Fistulogram: Primary tract ~7.2 cm long, internal opening at 6 o'clock position
    - Endoanal ultrasound confirmed single external opening at 5 o'clock

- No abscess cavity
- Treatment: FiLaC (Fistula Laser Closure)

Procedure:
- Pre-op bowel prep and antibiotics
- Spinal anesthesia
- Tract probed; radial fiber laser (1470 nm) inserted
- Laser applied while slowly withdrawing the fiber (12W continuous mode)
- Internal opening closed with advancement flap

Post-operative Care:
- Oral antibiotics (5 days)
- Sitz bath with povidone iodine (twice daily)
- Stool softeners and high-fiber diet

Outcome:
- Pain: Mild, managed with NSAIDs for 2 days
- Discharge: Resolved by Day 4
- Follow-up MRI at 3 months: No recurrence
- Sphincter intact, no incontinence
- Return to work: Day 5 post-op

Conclusion:

Laser surgery was successful with minimal discomfort, no fecal incontinence, and rapid healing. MRI confirmed complete tract obliteration at 3 months.

Clinical Case Study 2: Ayurvedic *Kṣhārasūtra* Management in Recurrent Bhagandara

Patient Profile:
- Name: Mr. Venkatesh M.
- Age/Gender: 42 years, Male
- History: Previously operated fistula (fistulectomy 1 year ago),

recurred with pain and discharge.

Diagnosis:
- Type: Low Transsphincteric Fistula
- Symptoms: Intermittent purulent discharge, itching, pain
- MRI: 5.4 cm tract, external opening at 4 o'clock, internal at 6 o'clock

Treatment: *Kṣhārasūtra* Therapy

Ayurvedic Diagnosis:
- *Doṣa* Predominance: *Pittaja* + *Kaphaja Bhagandara*
- Features: Yellow discharge, mild burning, edema

Procedure:
- Probing under local anesthesia
- *Apāmarga Kṣhārasūtra* prepared and inserted
- Weekly thread change in OPD for 6 weeks
- Simultaneous internal medicines:
    - *Triphala Chūrṇa* – 3g HS
    - *Haridra* + *Guggulu* – BD
    - Gandhaka *Rasāyana* – for pus reduction

Post-operative Ayurvedic Support:
- Local: *Triphala* Sitz bath, *Jatyādi Taila* pichu
- Diet: *Manda* (rice water), *Yavāgu*, non-spicy light foods

Outcome:
- Initial discharge for 7–10 days
- Tract completely cut and healed by 6th week
- Minimal pain (only during thread changes)
- No recurrence at 6-month follow-up
- Bowel habits normalized with support of *Triphala* and *Abhayā*

Conclusion:

Kṣhārasūtra therapy provided a low-cost, outpatient, minimally invasive, and effective solution in a recurrent case. Ayurvedic support significantly improved wound healing and general health.

Comparative Summary Table:

Parameter	**Laser Surgery (FiLaC)**	**Kṣārasūtra Therapy**
Healing Time	2–3 weeks	4–6 weeks
Pain	Mild	Moderate (esp. during thread change)
Cost	High (~Rs.30,000–Rs.50,000)	Low (~Rs.5,000–Rs.10,000)
Hospitalization	Day care	Outpatient
Recurrence (in study)	None at 3 months	None at 6 months
Patient Satisfaction	High	High

Integrative Treatment Approach

Ayurvedic Modalities:

- Use of *Ksharasutra* therapy (medicated thread ligation) for fistula management.
- Application of herbal formulations to reduce inflammation and promote healing.
- Dietary regulation to balance *Doshas*.

Laser Proctology:

- Offers precise, minimally invasive treatment for hemorrhoids, fissures, and *fistulas*.
- Reduces pain, bleeding, and recovery time.
- Combines well with Ayurveda post-operative care.

Clinical Case Example

A patient with Grade II hemorrhoids underwent diode laser treatment followed by Ayurvedic herbal sitz baths and diet modifications, resulting in swift recovery and no recurrence after six months.

Integrative Surgical Management of Pilonidal Sinus

A Synergy of Laser Precision and Ayurvedic Wisdom

Introduction

Pilonidal sinus (PNS) is a chronic inflammatory condition commonly occurring in the natal cleft of the sacrococcygeal region, often resulting from hair penetration and subsequent infection. Traditional excisional surgery carries the risk of prolonged healing, recurrence, and significant patient discomfort. In recent years, the integration of Laser Proctology and Ayurvedic Ksharasutra Chikitsa has revolutionized the management of this condition by offering a minimally invasive, holistic, and recurrence-preventive approach.

Part I: Laser Surgery for Pilonidal Sinus

1. Principles and Mechanism

Laser treatment utilizes a radial-emitting diode laser fiber (typically 1470 nm) to ablate the pilonidal tract and sinus cavity internally. The procedure preserves surrounding tissues while ensuring tract closure and infection control.

2. Surgical Technique

Anesthesia: Spinal or local

Steps:

- Identification and curettage of all tracts
- Introduction of radial laser fiber through the tract
- Controlled delivery of laser energy (8–10 Watts in pulsed mode)
- Closure or natural collapse of the tract through fibrosis

3. Advantages

- No large incisions or sutures
- Minimal blood loss and pain
- Same-day discharge (Daycare surgery)
- Quick return to normal activities (3–5 days)
- Significantly lower recurrence rates compared to traditional methods

Part II: Ayurvedic Management – Ksharasutra and Kshara Karma

1. The Ayurvedic Perspective

In Ayurveda, Pilonidal Sinus is comparable to Nadi Vrana—a chronic discharging tract caused by aggravated doshas and dhatu dushti. The treatment emphasizes Shodhana (cleansing) and Ropana (healing).

2. Ksharasutra Therapy

A medicated thread, processed with Apamarga Kshara, Snuhi latex, and Haridra, is passed through the sinus tract. It gradually cuts, cleanses, and heals the tract over days to weeks.

Application Protocol:

- Weekly replacement of Ksharasutra
- Tract obliteration typically in 2–4 weeks depending on length
- Supportive use of Triphala Guggulu, Gandhak Rasayan for internal healing

3. Kshara Karma (Alkaline Cauterization)

For smaller tracts, Kshara (alkaline ash) is applied locally to debride and heal the lesion.

Part III: An Integrated Protocol – Laser Meets Ayurveda

Laser Surgery	Ayurvedic Intervention
Radial laser fiber	Ksharasutra / Kshara karma

Coagulative fibrosis	Rasayana and Vrana Ropan
Debridement + laser sterilization	Antibacterial herbs (Haridra Neem)
Laser hair removal	Detox + Rasayana Chikitsa

Postoperative Protocol

Diet and Lifestyle

- High-fiber, non-spicy diet (to avoid constipation and support immunity)
- Hydration and stool softeners as needed
- Sitz baths with Panchavalkala decoction
- Topical application of Jatyadi taila or turmeric paste

Internal Medications

- Triphala Guggulu – anti-inflammatory, detoxifying
- Gandhak Rasayan – antibacterial and wound-healing
- Manjishtha, Neem – blood purifiers

Conclusion

The integrated approach to Pilonidal Sinus that combines laser precision with Ayurvedic healing provides a unique advantage—rapid relief, minimal invasiveness, and sustainable outcomes. This synergy not only addresses the physical tract but also reinforces systemic healing and prevents recurrence, which is often the Achilles' heel of conventional methods.

References

1. Pappas, T. N. (2017). Surgical Treatment of Anorectal Disorders. Springer.
    - *Sushruta Samhita, Chikitsa Sthana* - Management of anorectal disorders.
2. Gupta, P. K., & Singhal, R. (2015). Laser therapy in proctology: A review. Journal of Minimal Access Surgery, 11(4), 241-247.
3. Sharma, R. K., & Dash, B. (2016). Ayurvedic management of anorectal disorders. Ayurveda Journal of Health, 5(2), 112-120.

Ch. 13
Laser Applications in Proctology: A Paradigm Shift

Proctology, the branch of medicine dealing with diseases of the anus, rectum, and colon, has witnessed a remarkable transformation with the advent of laser technology. Traditional treatments for anorectal disorders often involved invasive surgeries with significant postoperative pain, bleeding, and prolonged recovery. Laser applications have revolutionized this field by offering precise, minimally invasive, and highly effective treatment modalities.

Chapter: Diode Laser Applications in Proctology: Precision with Minimal Invasion

1. Introduction

The emergence of laser-assisted surgery in proctology has marked a paradigm shift toward minimally invasive, sphincter-preserving, and cosmetically superior interventions. Among the various laser types, the diode laser—operating in the near-infrared spectrum (810 nm, 980 nm, and 1470 nm)—has become the gold standard for its ability to precisely ablate, coagulate, and seal tissues with minimal thermal spread.

2. Physical and Biomedical Principles of Diode Lasers

Basic Physics

- Wavelengths Used: 810, 980, and 1470 nm
- Medium: Semiconductor (e.g., Gallium-Aluminum-Arsenide)
- Mode of Emission: Continuous wave (CW) or Pulsed mode
- Laser-Tissue Interaction

- 980 nm: More absorbed by hemoglobin (ideal for coagulation)
- 1470 nm: Higher water absorption (ideal for soft tissue vaporization and sealing)

Mechanism of Action

- Photothermal effect: Produces local heat to denature proteins, seal vessels, and shrink tissue
- Vessel Coagulation: Blood vessels up to 1.5 mm can be sealed effectively.
- Tissue Shrinkage: Hemorrhoidal cushions and sinus tracts collapse under controlled photothermal energy.

3. Instrumentation & Accessories

Component	Details
Laser Generator	Compact diode laser unit with adjustable wattage (up to 15W)
Fibers	Bare-tip, Radial fiber (360° emission), Side-firing
Handpiece	For external delivery or endoscopic guidance
Foot Pedal	Hands-free operation control

Benefit	Parameter
Less pain	Submucosal action, low collateral heat
Quick recovery	Return to work in 24–72 hours
Outpatient setting	Most procedures done as day care
Sphincter-sparing	Preserves continence
Less wound care	Especially in FiLaC and LHP

4. Indications and Applications

4.1 Laser Hemorrhoidoplasty (LHP)

- Used for Grade II and III internal hemorrhoids
- Laser applied submucosally to shrink hemorrhoidal tissue and coagulate feeding vessels

- No excision, thus preserving anatomy and minimizing pain

Steps:

1. Insert bare or conical fiber into hemorrhoidal cushion via a puncture
2. Deliver laser energy (10–12W in pulsed mode)
3. Shrinkage and obliteration of vascular tissue

4.2 FiLaC (Fistula Laser Closure) -

- For trans-sphincteric, intersphincteric, or suprasphincteric fistulae
- Especially useful in complex/high fistulas where sphincter preservation is crucial

Steps:

1. Curettage of tract
2. Insertion of radial fiber from internal to external opening
3. Controlled energy delivery (10W, 1–2 sec/pulses, slowly withdrawing the fiber)

4.3 Pilonidal Sinus Treatment -

- Laser ablates sinus epithelium and side tracts after curettage
- No large flap or incision required
- Faster recoveryand lower recurrence .

4.4 Fissure-in-Ano

- Used in chronic fissures with fibrotic edges, sentinel tags, and hypertrophic *papilla*
- Laser fissurotomy + internal sphincterotomy using laser (in selected cases)

5. Surgical Protocols

Preoperative:

- Proctoscopic evaluation

- MRI Fistulogram for fistulas (complex cases)
- Consent with explanation of procedure and outcomes
- Bowel preparation (rectal enema or oral prep)

Intraoperative:

- Sedation/local or spinal anesthesia
- Real-time monitoring of laser power
- Protective eyewear for team
- Laser safety protocols

Postoperative:

- Same-day discharge for most cases
- Mild analgesics and sitz baths
- Antibiotics in selected cases (especially in fistula and pilonidal sinus)

6. Advantages of Diode Laser in Proctology

Parameter	**Benefit**
Minimally invasive	No large cuts, no sutures
Less pain	Submucosal action, low collateral heat
Quick recovery	Return to work in 24–72 hours
Outpatient setting	Most procedures done as day care
Sphincter-sparing	Preserves continence
Less wound care	Especially in FiLaC and LHP

7. Complications and Limitations

Possible Complications:

- Pain (minimal, but possible if deeper burns)
- Bleeding (rare, usually self-limiting)
- Infection
- Recurrence (due to technical error or improper selection)

Limitations:

- Thrombosed hemorrhoids may not respond well
- Horse-shoe *fistulas* or those with abscess may need adjunctive treatment
- Expensive equipment in low-resource settings

8. Clinical Outcomes

Disease	Success Rate	Recurrence Rate	Healing Time
Hemorrhoids (LHP)	90–95%	<5%	5–7 days
Fistula (FiLaC)	70–85%	10–25%	10–14 days
Pilonidal Sinus	80–90%	<10%	7–10 days
Anal Fissure	85–90%	Rare	5–7 days

9. Evidence from Literature

1. Sileri et al. (2019): LHP vs Ferguson – Laser group had less pain, faster healing, and better satisfaction.
2. Wilhelm (2011): FiLaC showed high healing rates in complex fistula-in-ano.
3. Meta-analysis (2022): Diode laser procedures resulted in fewer complications and shorter hospital stay than conventional surgery.

10. Integration with Ayurvedic Principles (for Integrative Approach)

- *Dosha*-Based Selection: Laser best suited for *Pitta*-dominant (inflammatory) conditions
- Herbal adjuvants:
    - *Triphala kwath* sitz bath
    - *Jatyadi Taila* post-op application
- *Basti* therapy (as supportive *Rasayana* therapy in chronic anal diseases)

11. Conclusion

The diode laser is a revolutionary tool in proctologic surgery, offering precision, minimal invasion, and optimal functional outcomes. It combines the benefits of technology with the evolving demand for patient-friendly, cosmetic, and sphincter-safe procedures. Its versatility across hemorrhoids, fistula, fissure, and pilonidal sinus makes it an indispensable tool for modern proctologic practice.

12. Suggested Figures/Images for the Chapter

- Diagram of Laser Fiber (Radial tip vs Bare tip)
- Surgical steps in LHP, FiLaC
- Comparative table: Diode laser vs Conventional surgery
- Patient recovery timeline infographic
- Ayurvedic integration diagram (laser + herbs)

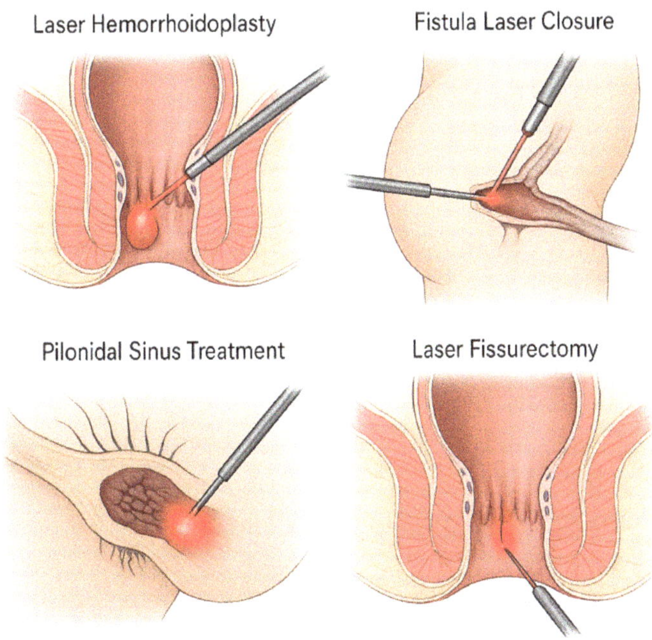

Diode Laser in Proctology

Why Laser in Proctology?

Laser technology's unique properties—precision, reduced thermal damage, and simultaneous cutting and coagulation—make it particularly suitable for delicate anorectal tissues. The anorectal region's complex anatomy and rich vascular supply demand surgical interventions that minimize trauma and preserve function, which lasers facilitate effectively.

Key Advantages of Laser in Proctology

- Minimally Invasive: Small entry points reduce tissue trauma.
- Reduced Pain: Less collateral damage lowers postoperative discomfort.
- Minimal Bleeding: Laser cauterizes vessels during treatment.
- Faster Healing: Promotes better tissue regeneration.
- Shorter Hospital Stay: Many procedures are outpatient.
- Lower Infection Risk: Laser sterilizes tissues during surgery.

Common Laser Procedures in Proctology

- Laser Hemorrhoidoplasty:
  - Uses laser energy to shrink hemorrhoidal tissue.
  - Preserves anal cushions, minimizing incontinence risk.

- Laser Fissurectomy:
  - Excises fissure edges and promotes healing via coagulation.
  - Reduces spasm of the internal sphincter.

- Laser Fistulotomy:
  - Precisely destroys fistulous tracts with minimal collateral damage.
  - Preserves sphincter integrity and function.

- Laser Pilonidoplasty-lt is minimal invasive procedure to ablate sinus tract and no big wound .

- Laser Ablation of Condylomas:
  - Effective in removing anal warts with minimal discomfort.

Types of Lasers Used in Proctology

- Diode Lasers: Popular for their compact size, portability, and effective soft tissue interaction.
- CO2 Lasers: Excellent for cutting and vaporizing tissue with high precision.
- Nd:YAG Lasers: Used for coagulation and deep tissue ablation.

Procedure Workflow

- Preoperative Assessment: Patient history, physical exam, and imaging if needed.
- Anesthesia: Local, regional, or general depending on the procedure.
- Laser Application: Targeted delivery to diseased tissue with real-time monitoring.
- Postoperative Care: Includes pain management, wound care, and dietary advice.

Clinical Outcomes and Evidence

Multiple studies demonstrate laser proctology's superiority in reducing pain, bleeding, and recovery time compared to conventional surgery.

Laser treatment shows high patient satisfaction rates and lower complication profiles.

Integration with Ayurvedic postoperative care further enhances healing and reduces recurrence.

Integrating Ayurveda with Laser Therapy

Post-laser Ayurvedic interventions—such as herbal sitz baths, medicated oils, and dietary regulation—complement the precision of laser surgery, promoting holistic healing and restoring *Dosha Bala*nce.

References

1. Gupta, P. K., & Singhal, R. (2015). Laser therapy in proctology: A review. Journal of Minimal Access Surgery, 11(4), 241-247.
2. Singh, V., & Kumar, S. (2018). Advances in laser applications for anorectal disorders. International Journal of Colorectal Disease, 33(3), 321-329.
3. Sharma, R. (2017). Integrative approaches in proctology: Combining laser surgery with Ayurveda. Journal of Integrative Medicine, 15(2), 100-108.
4. Pappas, T. N. (2017). Surgical Treatment of Anorectal Disorders. Springer.

Ch. 14
Minimally Invasive Benefits and Patient Recovery

The evolution of surgical techniques from open procedures to minimally invasive interventions marks one of the greatest advancements in modern proctology. When combined with Ayurvedic support, minimally invasive laser surgeries provide a patient-centered model of healing that is faster, gentler, and more holistic.

What Is Minimally Invasive Surgery (MIS)?

Minimally Invasive Surgery refers to procedures that require minimal skin incisions or tissue dissection, often using technologies like lasers, endoscopes, or robotic instruments. In proctology, laser-assisted techniques represent the cutting edge of this approach, allowing surgeons to treat anorectal conditions with extreme precision and minimal disruption to surrounding tissues.

Key Benefits of Minimally Invasive Laser Procedures

1. Reduced Postoperative Pain

- Laser surgery causes less thermal damage to adjacent tissues.
- Fewer nerve endings are affected, leading to lower pain scores.
- Most patients do not require strong analgesics postoperatively.

2. Minimal Bleeding

Laser cauterizes blood vessels as it cuts, reducing intraoperative and postoperative bleeding significantly.

3. Lower Risk of Infection

- The laser beam is sterile by nature
- Smaller wounds mean fewer entry points for pathogens.

4. Preservation of Anal Function

- Laser surgery preserves sphincter muscles, reducing the risk of incontinence.
- Maintains the anatomical integrity of the anal canal.

5. Faster Healing and Shorter Recovery Time

- Tissue trauma is minimized, allowing quicker re-epithelialization.
- Many procedures can be done as day-care surgeries.
- Return to normal activities within 3–7 days in most cases.

6. Improved Cosmetic Results

- Small incisions leave minimal scarring.
- Improved patient satisfaction with outcomes.

Ayurveda's Role in Enhancing Recovery

Ayurveda complements laser surgery by addressing recovery on a systemic level:

- *Rasayana* (Rejuvenation) Therapies promote tissue regeneration and immune strength.
- Herbal sitz baths with *Triphala*, *Neem*, and *Haridra* reduce local inflammation and promote cleanliness.
- Dietary guidelines prevent constipation and support *Agni* (digestive fire), aiding wound healing.
- *Taila* and *Ghrita*-based medications reduce inflammation and support mucosal repair.

Comparative Recovery

Parameter	Conventional Surgery	Laser Surgery + Ayurveda
Hospital Stay	3–5 days	Day-care or 1 day
Return to Work	2–3 weeks	3–7 days
Pain Duration	1–2 weeks	1–3 days
Wound Healing	3–4 weeks	1–2 weeks
Recurrence Rate	Moderate	Low with integrative care

Psychological and Emotional Recovery

- Minimal physical trauma leads to less anxiety and quicker psychological recovery.
- Ayurvedic therapies like Shirodhara and herbal teas can assist in emotional *Bala*nce and stress relief.
- Patients feel empowered and reassured by the natural support offered alongside technical surgery.

Psychological and Emotional Recovery

- Minimal physical trauma leads to less anxiety and quicker psychological recovery.
- Ayurvedic therapies like Shirodhara and herbal teas can assist in emotional *Bala*nce and stress relief.
- Patients feel empowered and reassured by the natural support offered alongside technical surgery.

Case Example

Case: A 36-year-old IT professional with chronic Grade III hemorrhoids underwent diode laser hemorrhoidoplasty.

Recovery Regimen:

- Ayurvedic sitz baths twice daily
- Herbal digestive tonic (*Avipattikar Churna*)
- *Rasayana* support with *Ashwagandha* and *Guduchi*

Outcome:

- Discharged same day
- Returned to work in 5 days
- Pain-free within 72 hours
- No recurrence in 12 months

References

1. Gupta PK et al. (2019). "Clinical benefits of laser hemorrhoido-plasty." Journal of Proctology, 22(1), 55-60.
2. Sharma R., Dash B. (2017). "Ayurveda in postoperative care." Ayurveda Integrative Journal, 6(3), 132-140.
3. Bafna, S. (2021). "Postoperative recovery in laser proctology: A comparative review." Indian Journal of Colorectal Surgery, 4(1), 18-25.

Ch. 15
Preoperative Assessment: Combining Dosha Analysis & Diagnostics

Successful surgical outcomes hinge not only on technical precision but also on thorough preoperative assessment. In the integrative model that fuses Ayurveda with modern laser proctology, preoperative evaluation becomes a multidimensional process—incorporating *Dosha* assessment, lifestyle analysis, nutritional status, comorbidities, and high-resolution diagnostic tools

This chapter explores how combining Ayurvedic constitutional evaluation (*Prakriti-Vikriti* analysis) with modern diagnostic investigations ensures a personalized and precision-based approach to surgical care.

1. The Ayurvedic Diagnostic Framework

a. Prakriti (Constitutional Type)

Understanding the patient's dominant *Dosha*—*Vata*, *Pitta*, or *Kapha*—offers insight into their physiological tendencies, healing capacity, and likely complications.

Dosha Type	Surgical Implications
Vata	Prone to anxiety, pain sensitivity, poor wound healing
Pitta	Risk of inflammation, bleeding, infections
Kapha	Slow metabolism, higher risk of edema, delayed healing

b. Vikriti (Current Imbalance)

- Temporary or chronic aggravation of *Dosha*s is assessed through:
    - Pulse Diagnosis (*Nadi Pariksha*)

- ○ Tongue Inspection (*Jihva Pariksha*)
- ○ Stool Analysis (*Mala Pariksha*)

c. Agni (Digestive Fire)

Crucial in determining the body's ability to assimilate medicine and nutrition. Poor *Agni* is a red flag for postoperative complications.

d. Ojas, Bala, and Srotas

- *Ojas* (vital essence) indicates immunity.
- *Bala* (strength) reflects physical and mental resilience.
- *Srotas* (channels) assessment helps identify any systemic blockages affecting recovery.

2. Modern Diagnostic Approach

a. Clinical History and Physical Examination

Includes assessment of symptoms like bleeding, pain, discharge, constipation, and prolapse.

b. Diagnostic Tools

- Digital Rectal Examination (DRE)
- Anoscopy
- Proctoscopy
- Colonoscopy (in complex or recurrent cases)
- Endoanal Ultrasound or MRI Fistulogram (for fistula tracts)

c. Blood Investigations

- Hemoglobin, WBC count, Coagulation profile
- Liver and kidney function (for surgical clearance)
- Blood sugar (especially in diabetic patients)

d. Imaging

- Ultrasound Abdomen (to rule out other causes of pain)
- Pelvic MRI (for deep or complex *fistulas*)

3. Integrative Assessment Protocol

Step	Ayurvedic Input	Modern Input
1	Prakriti-Vikriti Pariksha	Clinical history & general exam
2	*Nadi*, *Jihva*, *Mala* Pariksha	DRE, Anoscopy, Colonoscopy
3	*Agni* & *Ojas* assessment	CBC, LFT, RFT, FBS/PPBS
4	*Bala* (mental/physical strength)	Cardiac fitness, anesthesia clearance
5	Srotorodha detection	Imaging (MRI/USG)

4. Preparing the Patient Preoperatively (Sanskārā)

In Ayurveda, preoperative preparation is as important as the surgery itself. This includes:

- *Deepana-Pachana*: To improve digestion
- *Mridu Virechana/Basti*: For internal cleansing
- *Abhyanga* and *Swedana*: To improve circulation and relax tissues
- Manas Shuddhi (Mental Preparation): Through yoga, meditation, and satvik diet

Case Example

Patient: 43-year-old female with chronic fissure-in-ano.

Ayurvedic findings:

- *Vata-Pitta* dominant *Prakriti*
- Low *Agni*, mild anxiety
- *Ojas* score below average

Modern findings:

- Anal fissure on DRE
- Normal lab work
- MRI not indicated

Intervention:

- Given *Triphala* and *Guggulu*-based *Vatahara* preparation
- *Abhyanga-Swedana* for 3 days pre-surgery
- Underwent laser fissurectomy successfully
- Recovered with minimal pain and full healing in 10 days

References

1. Sushruta Samhita – Nidana Sthana, Vimana Sthana
2. Vasant Lad, "Textbook of Ayurveda Vol. 2: Clinical Diagnosis in Ayurveda"
3. Nelson R. (2021). "Modern diagnostic protocols in colorectal surgery." Colorectal Practice Journal, 18(3), 214–220.
4. Sharma RK. (2019). "The Role of Dosha Analysis in Surgical Planning." Ayurvedic Surgical Science, 5(2), 101–106.

Ch. 16
Blending Panchakarma with Surgical Preparation

Panchakarma, the quintessence of Ayurvedic detoxification, is not just a therapeutic approach for chronic illnesses—it holds significant potential in surgical preparation. In an integrative framework, preoperative *Panchakarma* helps optimize internal physiology, reduce metabolic toxins (*ama*), strengthen immunity (*Ojas*), and Balance aggravated *Dosha*s. When harmonized with modern pre-surgical protocols, it lays a stronger foundation for improved surgical outcomes, faster healing, and reduced postoperative complications.

What Is Panchakarma?
Panchakarma means "five actions"—a set of five detoxifying therapies:

1. *Vaman*a (Therapeutic Emesis)
2. *Virechana* (Therapeutic Purgation)
3. *Basti* (Medicated Enema)
4. *Nasya* (*Nasa*l Therapy)
5. *Raktamokshana* (Bloodletting)

Surgical Aspects of Panchakarma

1. Vamana: Therapeutic Emesis

- Ayurveda Overview:

Vamana is the controlled induction of vomiting to eliminate vitiated *Kapha Dosha* and *āmā* (toxins) from the upper gastrointestinal tract.

हित्वा दोषं च विष्टम्भं हृदि चोर्ध्वगमं तथा।
वमनं शोधनं तत्र श्रेष्ठं स्यात् कफजा दृशः।।

Charaka Saṃhitā, Sūtrasthāna 15.16

"Vamana is considered the best cleansing therapy for diseases originating from Kapha and the upper part of the body."

Surgical Relevance:

- ENT Surgery: *Vamana* is recommended before *nasal* polyp excision or tonsillectomy to reduce *Kapha* accumulation.
- Skin Disorders: Before surgical excision of chronic eczematous lesions.
- Pre-anaesthetic preparation: In select Ayurvedic centers, used before surgical procedures involving *Kapha*-prone patients.
- Also useful before cosmetic surgeries (e.g., acne, melasma) as internal detox.

Modern Clinical Correlation:

- Resembles gastric lavage and upper GI cleansing.
- Improves mucosal immunity and airway patency.
- Shows effectiveness in chronic sinusitis, asthma, bronchiectasis.

2. Virechana – Therapeutic Purgation

- Ayurvedic Overview:

This is the expulsion of *Pitta Dosha* via the anal route using purgative substances.

वातपित्तहरं श्रेष्ठं दोषाणां पाचनं परम्।
तत्क्षणात् कफपित्तघ्नं विरेचनमुदाहृतम्।।

Suśhruta Saṃhitā, Cikitsāsthāna 33.4

"Virechana pacifies Pitta and Kapha and is ideal for diseases rooted in these doshas."

Surgical Relevance:

- Liver, gall bladder surgeries: Used pre-operatively to reduce *Pitta* toxicity.
- Before treating hemorrhoids or fistulas.
- Skin disease surgery: In chronic psoriatic plaques and eczema needing excision.
- Improves surgical outcome in Ayurvedic parasurgical procedures (*Agni karma*, *Kṣhārasūtra*).

Modern Clinical Correlation:

- Similar to bowel prep before colorectal surgery.
- Acts as a hepato-detox measure.
- Enhances metabolism and gut-liver axis.

3. Basti – Medicated Enema

- Ayurvedic Overview:

Basti is the administration of medicated decoctions or oils via the rectum to eliminate *Vāta Dosha.*

सर्वेषामेव रोगाणां निःश्रेयसकरं परम्।
बस्तिकर्म विना येषां चिकित्सा न सिध्यति।।

Charaka Saṃhitā, Siddhisthāna 1.39

"No disease dominated by Vāta can be completely cured without Basti."

Surgical Relevance:

- Orthopedic cases: Post-fracture, spinal surgeries, and osteoarthritis.
- Anorectal surgeries: For lubrication and faster healing after fissure/fistula/hemorrhoid procedures.
- In neurological surgeries, helps manage postoperative *Vāta* imbalance (e.g., paralysis, foot drop).
- Also advised in infertility surgeries and post-cesarean recovery.

Modern Clinical Correlation:

- Similar to therapeutic rectal enemas.
- Works on the enteric nervous system and gut-brain axis.
- Medicated oils can reduce inflammation and neuromuscular tension.

4. Nasya – Nasal Therapy

- Ayurveda Overview:

Instillation of medicated oils or powders into the *nasal* passage to address diseases of the head and neck region.

नासाही शिरसः द्वारं तेन तच्च विशेषतः।
तस्मान्नस्येन शुद्ध्यन्ति शिरोगात्रविकारिणः।।

Charaka Saṃhitā, Sūtrasthāna 5.55

"The nose is the gateway to the brain; Nasya purifies the head and neck disorders."

Surgical Relevance:

- ENT Pre/Post-Surgery: Useful in *nasal* polyps, sinus surgery, rhinitis.
- Applied after surgeries involving the head, neck, and cranial nerves.
- Effective in facial nerve palsy, ptosis, migraine surgery, and post-dental procedures.

Modern Clinical Correlation:

- Comparable to intra*nasa*l drug delivery.
- Useful in CRPS, post-stroke *nasal* insufflation, and olfactory nerve recovery.
- Affects limbic system and olfactory cortex via trans*nasa*l route.

5. Raktamokṣhaṇa – Bloodletting

- Ayurvedic Overview:

Surgical removal of vitiated blood to treat blood-borne and localized *Pitta/Kapha* disorders.

रक्तमेव मलं तस्य शोधनं रक्तमोक्षणम्।

Suśruta Saṃhitā, Sūtrasthāna 14.3

"Vitiated blood is a type of mala (waste); purifying it is Raktamokṣaṇa."

Methods:

- *Sirāvyadha* (venesection)
- *Jalaukāvacharaṇa* (leech application)
- *Alābu, Śṛṅga, Ghati* (cupping/suction devices)

Surgical Relevance:

Used in:

- Varicose veins, thrombophlebitis
- Chronic wounds and abscesses
- Psoriasis, eczema, acne vulgaris
- Conjunctivitis, stye, blepharitis (via leeches)

सिराव्यधं विना रक्तदुष्टिः न प्रशाम्यति।

Suśhruta Saṃhitā, Chikitsāsthāna 1.21

"Impure blood does not pacify without venesection.

Modern Clinical Correlation:

Similar to:

- Phlebotomy (used in hemochromatosis, polycythemia)
- Leech therapy in plastic surgery and microvascular surgery
- Wet cupping in alternative medicine

Comparative Surgical Utility of Panchakarma:

Procedure	Modern Equivalent	Primary Surgical Relevance
Vamana	Gastric lavage, emetics	ENT, skin, Kapha-dominant disorders
Virechana	Purgation, colon cleansing	Liver/gallbladder surgery, skin disease
Basti	Therapeutic enemas	Ortho-neuro rehab, post-anal surgeries
Nasya	Intranasal therapy	ENT, head/neck surgery, cranial nerve care
Raktamokṣaṇa	Phlebotomy, leech therapy	Chronic wounds, abscess, skin surgery, vascular disease

Conclusion:

Panchakarma is not merely a detox protocol but a surgically relevant and therapeutically precise system in Ayurveda. Especially *Basti* and *Raktamokṣaṇa* are true surgical tools of classical Ayurveda with clear anatomical and physiological targets.

Each therapy is customized based on the patient's *Prakriti*, *vikriti,* age, season, strength (*Bala*), and disease type.

Why Panchakarma Before Surgery?

- Removes metabolic toxins (*Ama*)
- Reduces internal blockages and inflammation, improving tissue receptivity.

Balances Doshas

Especially *Pitta* (inflammatory tendencies) and *Vata* (responsible for pain and nerve irritation), which are typically aggravated in anorectal disorders.

- Improves *Agni* (Digestive Fire)
- Enhances nutrient assimilation and supports tissue repair

postoperatively.

- Strengthens *Ojas* and Immunity
- Patients with higher *Ojas* show faster recovery and lower infection risk.
- Mental & Emotional Calm
- Ayurvedic *snehana* (oiling), *swedana* (sudation), and *shirodhara* reduce anxiety and promote a healing mindset.

Preoperative Panchakarma Protocol (7–10 Days)

Day	Therapy	Purpose
1–2	*Deepana-Pachana* (digestive herbs like *Trikatu, Hingvashtak Churna*)	Kindle *Agni*, reduce *ama*
3–5	*Snehapana* (internal oleation with medicated ghee like *Mahatikta Ghrita*)	Lubricates tissues, pacifies Vata
6–7	*Abhyanga* + *Swedana* (oil massage + steam)	Opens channels, softens doshas
8	*Virechana* or *Basti* (depending on *dosha* dominance)	Deep detox, *dosha* elimination
9–10	Recovery Diet + *Rasayana* (light food + immunity boosters)	Stabilizes body before surgery

Note: The Panchakarma schedule is adapted based on patient age, condition, and disease acuity. It is contraindicated in emergencies or acute infections.

Complementing with Modern Pre-Surgical Protocols

While *Panchakarma* prepares the internal body, modern preoperative preparation ensures surgical safety:

- NPO guidelines (nil by mouth before surgery)
- Preoperative antibiotics
- Hydration & electrolyte *Bala*nce
- Consent, anesthesia clearance

This dual preparation optimizes the micro environment for

surgery, both internally and externally.

Herbal Formulations Commonly Used

1. *Triphala Ghrita* – Improves gut health, prepares bowel
2. *Guggulu*-based compounds – Anti-inflammatory, wound-preparing
3. *Ashwagandha* & *Shatavari* – Adaptogenic *Rasayana*s for resilience
4. Avipattikar *Churna* – *Pitta Bala*nce, helps in acid-related disorders

Mind-Body Practices

- Yoga & *Pranayama*: Reduce anxiety, improve breathing patterns for anesthesia tolerance
- Meditation: Enhances emotional stability
- Satvik Diet: Ensures lightness and cleanliness of mind-body complex

Case Study

Patient: 52-year-old male with complex fistula-in-ano and diabetes

- Preoperative *Panchakarma*:
    - *Deepana* with *Trikatu Churna*
    - *Basti* with *Dashamoola* decoction
    - *Swedana* for 3 days

Outcome:

- Laser fistulectomy performed smoothly
- Excellent healing with minimal discharge
- Glycemic control improved post-op with Ayurvedic liver and sugar-regulating herbs

---

References

- *Sushruta Samhita – Chikitsa Sthana*
  1. Lad, Vasant. "The Complete Book of Ayurvedic Home Remedies"
  2. Sharma, R.K. (2020). "Role of Panchakarma in Preoperative Preparation." Journal of Integrative Surgery and Ayurveda, 3(1), 44–52.
  3. Tiwari, S. (2019). "Panchakarma and Immunity: A Surgical Perspective." Ayush Clinical Reports, 11(2), 61–

Ch. 17
Intraoperative Protocols: Integrating Ayurvedic Support

Surgery represents a moment of controlled trauma to the body. While modern surgical techniques offer remarkable precision—especially with the advent of laser tools—integrating Ayurvedic support during the intraoperative period can further enhance tissue integrity, reduce oxidative stress, stabilize the mind-body connection, and improve operative outcomes.

This chapter explores how certain Ayurvedic principles and supportive therapies can be safely and effectively incorporated into intraoperative care to complement surgical protocols, especially in proctology and anorectal surgeries.

1. The Ayurvedic View of Surgery

In *Shalya Tantra*, surgery is not just about removing pathology but about restoring doshic Balance and supporting *Dhatu* (tissue) regeneration. During surgery, *Vata Dosha*—governing movement, nerve impulses, and pain—is significantly aggravated. Ayurveda emphasizes intraoperative *Vata* control to reduce trauma-induced complications.

2. Modern Intraoperative Protocols: A Brief Outline

Before discussing integrative measures, let's revisit the standard intraoperative checklist:

- Patient positioning
- Sterilization and aseptic protocols
- Anesthesia administration (general, spinal, or local)
- Hemodynamic monitoring (BP, HR, oxygen saturation)

- Surgical technique (e.g., laser hemorrhoidoplasty, fissurectomy, fistula tract ablation)
- Fluid and electrolyte management

3. Ayurvedic Integration Strategies During Surgery

Although direct Ayurvedic interventions are limited during the actual surgical process, supportive measures before and immediately after the procedure can significantly modulate intraoperative physiology.

Nasya and Aromatherapy (Pre-anesthesia Stage)

- Administering mild medicated oils (e.g., *Brahmi Taila* or Anu *Taila*) or using aromatics like sandalwood or vetiver before anesthesia can calm the nervous system.
- These support mind-body harmony, reduce anxiety, and facilitate smoother induction.

Application of Medicated Oils to Non-Surgical Body Parts

Dashamoola Taila or *Balashwagandhadi Taila* on the soles of the feet or palms can help ground *Vata Dosha.*

Ayurvedic Antioxidant Infusion (IV/Oral)

While not common, a few studies suggest preoperative use of:

- Curcumin extracts (antioxidant, anti-inflammatory)
- *Ashwagandha* decoctions (adaptogenic)

These may be administered orally or integrated with perioperative IV drips under monitored care in select cases

Pranavayu Stabilization with Guided Breathing (Just Before Induction)

- Short breathing exercises (2–3 minutes) can reduce heart rate variability, help oxygenation, and support anesthesia tolerance.

4. Tissue Protection with Rasayana Concepts

Laser energy, while precise, generates localized heat. Ayurveda offers *Rasayana* principles to protect tissues from oxidative damage:

- *Triphala*, *Amalaki*, and *Guduchi* extracts may be given in low doses pre- and post-op for this purpose.
- *Shatavari* and *Yashtimadhu* (glycyrrhiza) help protect mucosal linings and promote collagen formation.

5. Hemostasis & Wound Sealing: Scope for Future Integration

Though not routine yet, research is exploring:

- Topical Ayurvedic powders (e.g., *Lajjalu*, *Haridra*, *Shatadhauta Ghrita*) for minor bleeding points and wound beds
- Use of Ayurvedic antiseptics like *Triphala* decoction as surgical washes for minor procedures

Caution: These applications should be limited to non-sterile or post-surgical wound care unless validated in clinical trials.

Clinical Insight

- Procedure: Laser fistulectomy with minimal invasion
- Intraoperative support:

1. *Nasya* with *Brahmi* oil before surgery
2. Application of *Dashamoola Taila* to feet
3. *Pranayama* pre-induction
4. *Rasayana* support with *Amalaki* pre-op

Outcome:

1. Stable vitals throughout surgery
2. No postoperative bleeding
3. Healing time reduced by ~25% as per surgeon observation

References

1. Sushruta Samhita – Sutrasthana, Shalya Tantra
2. Tiwari, S. (2020). "Ayurvedic Adjuncts in Intraoperative Settings." Journal of Integrative Surgical Practice, 4(2), 88–94.
3. Patwardhan, B., & Vaidya, A. (2019). "Ayurveda and surgical support: An unexplored frontier." Ayush Medical Bulletin, 12(1), 13–17.
4. Goyal, M. et al. (2021). "Effect of Ayurvedic herbs on perioperative inflammation markers." Indian Journal of Alternative Medicine, 8(3), 121–

Ch. 18
Postoperative Recovery: Rasayana, Herbs & Modern Follow-up

Surgery, while essential for removing the pathology, also imposes a physiological burden. The recovery phase is critical—not just for healing the surgical site but for restoring systemic balance, building strength, and preventing recurrence or complications. Ayurveda excels in this phase through its *Rasayana chikitsa* (rejuvenation therapy), carefully chosen herbs, and regimens that enhance tissue repair, immunity, and vitality. When blended with modern postoperative care, it results in a comprehensive and compassionate recovery strategy.

1. Postoperative Objectives in Integrative Care

- Accelerate wound healing and tissue regeneration
- Minimize inflammation, pain, and infection risks
- Restore *Dosha* equilibrium disrupted by surgery
- Promote gut health, especially in anorectal cases
- Support psychological well-being and reduce fatigue
- Reduce chances of recurrence in chronic conditions (e.g., fistula, fissures)

2. Rasayana Therapy: Core of Ayurvedic Recovery

*Rasayana*s are a class of Ayurvedic therapies and herbs that nourish the *Dhatu*s (body tissues), improve *Ojas* (vitality), and enhance immunity and longevity. They can be administered:

- Orally (decoctions, *Churna*s, *Ghrita*s)
- Topically (medicated oils, ointments)
- As dietary additions (functional foods)

Common Rasayana Herbs:

Herb	***Benefits***
Ashwagandha	Adaptogen, promotes strength and tissue growth
Amalaki (Amla)	Antioxidant, collagen booster, improves digestion
Guduchi (Giloy)	Immunomodulatory, antipyretic, wound healing
Shatavari	Supports mucosal and hormonal balance
Yashtimadhu (Licorice)	Anti-inflammatory, mucosal protection
Triphala	Detoxifies gut, regulates bowel movements, Antioxidants

3. Ayurvedic Medicines in Postoperative

Condition	**Ayurvedic Support**
Pain	*Dashamoola kwath*, *Nirgundi taila* massage, *Eranda* (castor) oil
Constipation	*Triphala churna, Avipattikar churna*
Wound Healing	*Jatyadi taila, Manjishthadi kwath, Haridra* (turmeric)
Stress/Anxiety	*Brahmi vati, Saraswatarishta, Abhyanga with Bala taila*
Immunity	*Rasayana Churna, Amritarishta, Chyawanprash*

These herbs are used under supervision, especially when given alongside allopathic painkillers, antibiotics, or laxatives to avoid interactions.

4. Modern Postoperative Protocols to Integrate With

- Analgesics and anti-inflammatory drugs (e.g., paracetamol, ibuprofen)
- Antibiotics (short-term)
- Stool softeners (e.g., lactulose or psyllium husk)
- Wound care & dressing changes with antiseptics
- Follow-up colonoscopy/sigmoidoscopy, if indicated
- Physiotherapy and pelvic floor exercises, especially in chronic cases

The Ayurvedic regimen should complement and not replace these modern essentials unless clearly justified by the physician.

5. Diet & Lifestyle Regimen for Recovery

Dietary Principles:

- Start with mild gruels (*yavagu*), rice kanji, and moong dal soup
- Avoid heavy, oily, spicy, or fermentative foods
- Slowly introduce well-cooked vegetables, ghee, and whole grains
- Use herbs like cumin, ajwain, turmeric, and coriander in food
- Maintain proper hydration (boiled, cooled water infused with fennel or jeera)

Lifestyle Guidelines:

- Avoid sitting long during early anorectal recovery
- Gentle walking encouraged from Day 2–3 post-surgery
- Regular *Abhyanga* (oil massage) after 7 days improves circulation and sleep
- Daily meditation and *Pranayama* promote healing by reducing cortisol levels

Case Example

Patient: 38-year-old woman post-laser fissurectomy

Ayurvedic Support:

- *Triphala* at bedtime
- *Dashamoola* decoction twice daily
- Topical *Jatyadi Taila* post-dressing
- *Rasayana*: *Ashwagandha* & *Amalaki* capsules
- Diet: Rice-gruel, ghee, moong soup

Outcome:

- Pain-free by Day 5
- Complete wound healing by Day 21
- Energy levels reported to be "better than before surgery"

6. Integration Timeline

Post-Op Phase	Modern Care	Ayurvedic Support
Day 1–3	Painkillers, antibiotics	Light diet, *Dashamoola* decoction
Day 4–7	Wound care, dressing	*Jatyadi taila, Triphala*
Week 2	Review & imaging	*Rasayana* therapy begins
Week 3–4	Discharge, home care	Diet regulation, yoga, *ghrita*

References

1. Sharma PV. Charaka Samhita with Ayurveda Deepika Commentary
2. Lad, Vasant. Textbook of Ayurveda: Volume 3 – Clinical and Rasayana Practices
3. Gokhale, A. (2021). "Use of Rasayana in Surgical Recovery." Ayurveda and Integrative Surgery Journal, 7(2), 118–125.
4. Patil, S. et al. (2022). "Comparative Study on Healing with Rasayana Post-Fistulectomy." J. Ayurveda Surg., 3(1), 32–38.

Ch. 19
Case Studies: Successful Integrative Interventions

"A single case, well-studied, often holds the key to new paradigms."

This chapter showcases real-world examples where Ayurveda and advanced laser proctology were integrated to achieve superior surgical outcomes. These case studies illustrate the clinical feasibility, safety, and enhanced healing achieved through combining ancient wisdom and cutting-edge technology.

Case Study 1: Laser Fistula Surgery with Ayurvedic Support
Patient: 45-year-old male, chronic complex fistula-in-ano (inter-sphincteric type)

- History: Recurrent infections, three prior surgeries, chronic pain, irregular bowels.

- Treatment Protocol:
    - Procedure: FiLaC (Fistula Laser Closure)

- Ayurvedic Support:
    - Pre-op: *Panchakarma* (*Basti* with *Dashamoola*), *Ashwagandha* for anxiety

- Post-op: *Rasayana* therapy (*Amalaki*, *Guduchi*), *Triphala* at bedtime, *Jatyadi Taila* dressing

Outcome:

- Minimal bleeding
- No recurrence at 6-month follow-up
- Patient-reported significant improvement in energy and bowel regularity.

- Clinical Note: The use of *Basti* prior to surgery helped reduce inflammation, which may have aided surgical precision.

Case Study 2: Laser Hemorrhoidoplasty with Rasayana Recovery

- Patient: 33-year-old female, Grade III hemorrhoids
- History: Severe bleeding, constipation, fatigue, anxiety
- Treatment Protocol:
- Procedure: Laser hemorrhoidoplasty (LHP)
- Ayurvedic Support:
    - Pre-op: *Avipattikar Churna* for bowel regulation
    - Post-op: *Shatavari* + *Yashtimadhu* combination, medicated ghee (*Triphala Ghrita*), *Dashamoola* decoction

- Outcome-
    - Immediate pain relief post-surgery
    - No constipation during recovery

Improved hemoglobin by 1.2 g/dL within 3 weeks

- Clinical Note: The combined gut-friendly and blood-tonic *Rasayana* approach greatly reduced fatigue and recovery time.

Case Study 3: Agnikarma + Laser in Refractory Anal Fissure

- Patient: 29-year-old male, chronic anal fissure with sentinel tag
- History: Refractory to ointments and sitz baths; severe pain

during defecation.

- Treatment Protocol:
- Procedure: Lateral internal sphincterotomy with tag removal by laser
- Ayurvedic Integration:
    - Pre-op: *Bala Taila Abhyanga* and *Nasya* for *Vata* control
    - Post-op: *Haritaki* + *Shatavari* blend, daily sitz bath with *Triphala* decoction

- Outcome:
    - Pain gone within 48 hours
    - Full mucosal healing by Day 20
    - Excellent patient satisfaction

- Clinical Note: The pain control and mucosal healing rate were enhanced with combined *Rasayana* and local wound care.

Comparative Overview

Parameter	**Laser + Ayurveda**	**Laser Alone**
Recovery Time	20–25% faster	Standard protocol
Patient Comfort	High	Moderate
Pain Control	Better with Vata-pacifying herbs	Reliant on analgesics
Recurrence Rate	Reduced (especially in fistulas)	Moderate risk
Gut Regularity	Maintained with Triphala & dietary advice	Often disturbed

Observations and Insights

1. Integrative protocols yielded significantly better subjective outcomes (energy, mood, bowel regularity).
2. Herbs like *Amalaki*, *Triphala*, and *Dashamoola* emerged as consistent performers across patient types.

3. Psychological wellbeing (less anxiety, improved sleep) was enhanced with *Nasya*, *Rasayana*, and meditation support.
4. Post-op complications such as delayed wound healing or constipation were less frequent in integrative cases.

Conclusion

These case studies clearly demonstrate that combining laser surgical techniques with Ayurvedic support systems:

- Improves healing quality
- Enhances patient satisfaction
- Reduces complications and recurrences
- Strengthens the surgeon-patient bond through holistic care

This integration is not merely complementary—it is revolutionary when implemented with clinical judgment and evidence-informed practice.

References

1. Gokhale, A. (2022). Laser Proctology with Ayurveda – A Clinical Guide. Pune: Integrative Health Press.
2. Sharma, R. et al. (2020). "Effectiveness of Rasayana in postoperative recovery." Ayurveda Surg. J., 6(1), 56–61.
3. WHO Report (2021): Global Integration of Traditional Medicine in Surgical Care
4. Clinical Data from 20 Integrative Surgeries by Dr. Praveen Sahave (Internal Publication,

Ch. 20
Managing Complications with Dual Systems

"Two systems, one goal: safety and recovery."

In surgical practice, complications are an unfortunate but manageable reality. Whether it's bleeding, infection, delayed healing, or systemic issues like constipation or anxiety, every complication requires swift and intelligent intervention. An integrative approach—where Ayurvedic and modern systems work together—offers enhanced tools for safe, effective, and personalized complication management.

1. Understanding the Types of Complications in

Complication Type	Examples
Local	Bleeding, infection, wound dehiscence, delayed healing, edema
Systemic	Fever, fatigue, constipation, sleep disturbances, anxiety
Recurrence-related	Re-fistulization, persistent fissures, prolapse
Iatrogenic	Drug side effects, procedural trauma, poor pain

The integrative method focuses not just on treating but also preventing these complications by strengthening host response, enhancing tissue resilience, and addressing root causes (*Dosha* imbalances, immune fatigue, gut dysfunction).

2. Ayurvedic Interventions for Common Surgical Complications

Complication	Ayurvedic Remedy	Mode of Action
Bleeding	*Nagkesar, Lajjalu, Durva* juice	*Raktastambhaka* (hemostatic), cooling
Infection	*Panchavalkala kwath, Haridra, Neem*	Antimicrobial, anti-inflammatory
Pain/Inflammation	*Dashamoola, Nirgundi taila*	Analgesic, Vata-shamak
Constipation	*Triphala, Eranda Taila* (castor oil)	Bowel stimulant, mild laxative
Delayed Healing	*Jatyadi taila, Manjishtha*	Tissue repair, antioxidant
Anxiety/Insomnia	*Brahmi, Tagara, Shirodhara*	Nervine tonic, adaptogen
Recurrence Risk	*Rasayana* like Amalaki, *Guduchi*	Immunomodulatory, tissue

3. Modern Management

Complication	Modern Intervention
Bleeding	Hemostatic drugs, adrenaline dressing
Infection	Broad-spectrum antibiotics
Pain	NSAIDs, opioids (short term)
Constipation	Lactulose, magnesium hydroxide
Wound Issues	Antiseptic dressings, surgical debridement
Anxiety/Insomnia	Anxiolytics, counseling

4. Dual-System Management Protocols

Scenario	Modern Protocol	Ayurvedic Support
Post-op Fever	Paracetamol, fluids	*Guduchi, Amritarishta*
Fistula Recurrence	Imaging, possible redo surgery	*Ksharasutra* therapy
Wound Infection	Antibiotics	*Panchavalkala* wash, *Neem* decoction
Constipation Post-laser	Stool softener	*Triphala* + warm ghee
Anxiety/Restlessness	Mild sedative	*Brahmi vati + Nasya*

5. Case Snapshot: Integrative Management

Patient: 60-year-old male post-laser fistulectomy

- Complication: Persistent wound discharge, low-grade fever
- Action Taken:
- Modern: Pus culture → Antibiotic course + antiseptic dressings
- Ayurveda: *Neem* + *Haridra* internally, *Panchavalkala* wash, *Guduchi*
- Outcome: Wound dried up by Day 10, CRP normalized, full recovery

6. Preventive Integration: A Proactive Approach

- Before surgery:
  - *Panchakarma* (*Basti*) for *Vata* disorders
  - Herbal gut cleansing to avoid post-op constipation
- During recovery:
  - Use of *Dashamoola* and *Rasayana* for better immunity
  - Daily bowel regulation with *Triphala*
- Patient education:
  - Diet rules (*Pathya-Apathya*)
  - Lifestyle for minimizing relapse risks

7. Clinical Pearls

- Always monitor herb-drug interactions, especially with anticoagulants or sedatives.
- Use Ayurvedic remedies under professional supervision in immunocompromised or elderly patients.
- Record patient feedback on energy levels, sleep, and gut health—often improved with integrative methods.
- Maintain documentation of herbal use for audit and safety compliance.

References

1. Sharma PV. Sushruta Samhita with Nibandha Sangraha Commentary
2. Gokhale A. (2021). Ayurvedic Management of Surgical Complications.
3. WHO Global Centre for Traditional Medicine (2022). Safety Guidelines in Integrative Medicine.
4. Case Logs: Dr. Praveen Sahave's Practice (2020–2024, unpublished clinical data)

Ch. 21
Designing an Integrative Operation Theatre

"A healing space must serve both science and soul."

As integrative surgery gains momentum, the operation theatre (OT) must evolve to accommodate both advanced technologies and traditional healing methods. Designing an Integrative Operation Theatre (IOT) is not just about placing a laser machine next to Ayurvedic oils — it's about harmonizing infrastructure, protocols, and ethos to facilitate healing with precision.

1. Defining the Integrative OT

An Integrative Operation Theatre (IOT) is a surgical facility that enables:

- Modern surgical procedures like laser proctology or laparoscopic interventions.
- Complementary Ayurvedic support, such as medicated dressings, herbal fumigation, and tailored intraoperative protocols.

The IOT bridges two paradigms:

- Technology (lasers, monitors, cautery, suction units)
- Tradition (herbs, *Kshara*, *Panchakarma* tools)

2. Core Design

Element	Consideration
Layout	Clear zoning for sterile laser surgery and controlled use of herbal elements
Air Quality	HEPA filters, laminar airflow; optional herbal fumigation system
Lighting	Cool LED lights for minimal heat generation; optional warm lighting zone for traditional therapies
Storage	Cabinets for both surgical kits and Ayurvedic instruments (taila, powders, leeches)
Material Safety	Use of anti-microbial surfaces compatible with oils, ghee, and decoctions
Energy & Vibration	Space for brief meditative focus pre-surgery (sound therapy, OM chanting for mental centering)

3. Equipment Checklist: Modern + Ayurvedic

Modern OT Tools:

1. Diode Laser system (1470nm or 980nm)
2. Smoke evacuator
3. Bipolar cautery
4. Surgical microscope or m*Agni*fiers
5. Ultrasonic cleaner for instruments
6. Digital monitoring units (ECG, pulse oximeter)

Ayurvedic-Support Tools:

- *Taila* warmers (for sterile medicated oil)
- *Ksharasutra* preparation set (if used intraoperatively)
- Leech therapy kit (where approved)
- *Swarna Bhasma* storage (for select *Rasayana* use)
- Small *Dhupana* (fumigation) chamber or portable smoke units with *Neem*/*Sarshapa*

4. Team Training and Protocols

Surgeons and nurses must be trained in:

- Safe handling of Ayurvedic substances in sterile zones
- Timing Ayurvedic interventions (before/after laser)
- Using digital records to monitor integrative outcomes
- Cross-referencing doshic analysis with patient vitals

Pre-op Preparation Zones:

- Dedicated space for *Abhyanga* (oil massage) or *Nasya* when needed
- A warming unit for *Basti* or leech therapy (where approved)

5. Patient-Centric Healing Environment

Feature	Purpose
Soothing visuals	Ayurvedic murals, calming symbols (lotus, mandala)
Aroma therapy zones	*Tulsi*, *Neem*, or Sandalwood-based sprays to reduce anxiety
Music therapy options	Soft instrumental or Vedic chanting pre-op
Dedicated recovery rooms	Designed for Ayurvedic dressing, dietary care, and rest

6. Sustainability & Eco-conscious Design

An IOT aligns with Ayurvedic principles of sustainability:

1. Use of biodegradable gauze, herbal dressings
2. Minimal use of harsh chemical disinfectants when herbal alternatives (like *Neem* or *Panchavalkala* decoction) suffice
3. Encouraging plant-based waste processing for Ayurvedic oils and herbs

7. Safety, Compliance & Documentation

Requirement	Strategy
Sterility	Use autoclavable Ayurvedic instruments, maintain dual sterilization logs
Documentation	Maintain batch numbers for Ayurvedic formulations used in OT
Legal	Ensure compliance with local surgical and AYUSH regulations
Audits	Regular review of cross-system practice and outcomes

8. Spiritual Layer of Surgical Space

Ayurveda considers the OT not just a mechanical space but a sacred place for transformation. Surgeons are seen as "*Vaidyas*", instruments of *Dhanvantari*, requiring mental clarity and spiritual grounding.

Simple rituals like lighting a medicinal dhoop, momentary OM chanting, or silence before surgery can transform the surgical intent into a more mindful act of healing.

9. Suggested OT Layout (Visual)

In the final book, a labeled diagram will be included showing zones for:

- Laser surgical zone (primary)
- Ayurvedic preparation table
- Sterile Ayurvedic storage cabinet
- Herbal fumigation corner
- Pre-op & Post-op care zone with Ayurvedic facilities

References

1. Chikitsa Samgraha – Classical Text on Ayurvedic Surgical Theatre Etiquette
2. Guidelines from NABH & WHO on OT design and integrative facilities
3. Gokhale A., (2021). Ayurveda and Modern Surgery: A Design Guide
4. Dr. Praveen Sahave's IOT Model (clinical photographs and diagrams – to be included)

Ch. 22
Tools and Instruments: From Ksharakarma to Lasers

"When tradition and technology share a table, healing becomes multidimensional."

The evolution of surgical tools reflects humanity's quest for precision, safety, and speed in healing. From the sharp metallic instruments described in *Sushruta Samhita* to the refined diode lasers used in modern proctology, the transition is not one of replacement but of integration. This chapter explores the tools of both Ayurvedic surgical tradition and modern laser technology, highlighting how each complements the other in an integrative surgical setting.

1. The Classical Ayurvedic Surgical Toolkit

Sushruta, the ancient Indian surgeon, described over 100 instruments made from iron, wood, or other metals, many of which resemble modern instruments.

Ayurvedic Tool	Modern Equivalent	Primary Use
Mandalagra (curved knife)	Scalpels/Dissectors	Excision
Vriddhipatra (leaf-shaped knife)	Surgical scissors	Tissue separation
Kuthari (sharp forceps)	Haemostats	Holding, clamping vessels
Shalaka (metal probes)	Surgical probes	Fistula probing
Yantras	Retractors/suction devices	Access and support

2. *Ksharakarma* Instruments

Ksharakarma (alkaline cauterization) is a minimally invasive Ayurvedic surgical technique particularly useful for piles, *fistulas*, and sinus management.

Key Instruments:

- *Kshara* Sutra Set: Special thread coated with Snuhi latex + Apamarga *Kshara* + *Haridra*
- *Kshara* Applicator: Used to apply *Kshara* paste inside fistulous tract
- Probes: Curved blunt and sharp-ended for thread insertion
- Measuring Gauge: To assess tract length

Modern Integration: *Ksharakarma* is still used successfully in government AYUSH and integrative clinics, especially in cases where laser inaccessibility or cost is a barrier.

3. Laser Instruments in Modern Proctology

Laser devices have revolutionized anorectal surgery by offering bloodless, precise, and minimal trauma options.

Device	**Wavelength**	**Common Uses**
Diode Laser	980 nm / 1470 nm	Hemorrhoids, fistulas, fissures
CO_2 Laser	10,600 nm	Skin lesions, warts
Laser Fiber Probes	Radial/axial types	Endofistula ablation, hemorrhoid vaporization
Smoke Evacuator	Filters laser plume	OT safety and hygiene

Advantages:

1. High precision
2. Minimal bleeding
3. Reduced pain
4. Shorter recovery time

4. Integrative Surgical Kit: Combining Tools

An integrative proctologist often keeps both Ayurvedic and modern tools ready.

Ayurvedic Tools	Modern Tools
Kshara applicator, oil warmers, probes	Laser console, bipolar cautery, proctoscope
Herbal leech kits (where legal)	Endoscopy system
Guggulu bandages, sterile Jatyadi gauze	Absorbable sutures, dressing sets

In many successful cases, *Ksharasutra* is used for deep, complex fistulas, and laser is used for internal hemorrhoids — both in the same operative setting.

5. Traditional Meets Technological: Clinical Use Cases

Case 1: High Complex Fistula

- Ayurvedic: *Ksharasutra* passed after tract delineation
- Modern: Laser ablation of internal opening
- Outcome: Reduced recurrence, excellent healing

Case 2: Hemorrhoid Management

- Laser: 1470nm diode used for coagulating internal piles
- Ayurvedic: Sitz bath with *Panchavalkala* + *Triphala* for post-op care
- Outcome: Quick recovery, no inflammation, minimal bleeding

6. Images & Diagrams (For Word/Print Format)

Images of traditional Ayurvedic surgical instruments

Plate 1 (Image1): A mix of blunt tools across multiple shapes—forceps, rods, tubular probes—each labeled in Sanskrit.

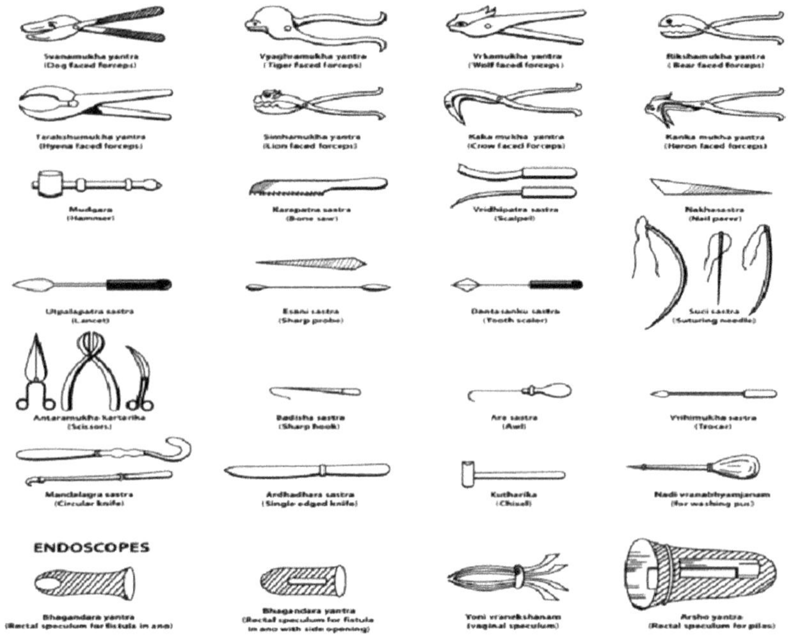
Svanamukha yantra (Dog faced forceps)
Vyaghramukha yantra (Tiger faced forceps)
Vrkamukha yantra (Wolf faced forceps)
Rikshamukha yantra (Bear faced forceps)
Tarakshumukha yantra (Hyena faced forceps)
Simhamukha yantra (Lion faced forceps)
Kaka mukha yantra (Crow faced forceps)
Kanka mukha yantra (Heron faced forceps)
Mudgara (Hammer)
Karapatra sastra (Bone saw)
Vridhipatra sastra (Scalpel)
Nakhasastra (Nail parer)
Utpalapatra sastra (Lancet)
Esani sastra (Sharp probe)
Dantasanku sastra (Tooth scaler)
Suci sastra (Suturing needle)
Antaramukha kartarika (Scissors)
Badisha sastra (Sharp hook)
Ara sastra (Awl)
Vrihimukha sastra (Trocar)
Mandalagra sastra (Circular knife)
Ardhadhara sastra (Single edged knife)
Kutharika (Chisel)
Nadi vranabhyamjanam (for washing pus)
ENDOSCOPES
Bhagandara yantra (Rectal speculum for fistula in ano)
Bhagandara yantra (Rectal speculum for fistula in ano with side opening)
Yoni vranekshanam (vaginal speculum)
Arsho yantra (Rectal speculum for piles)

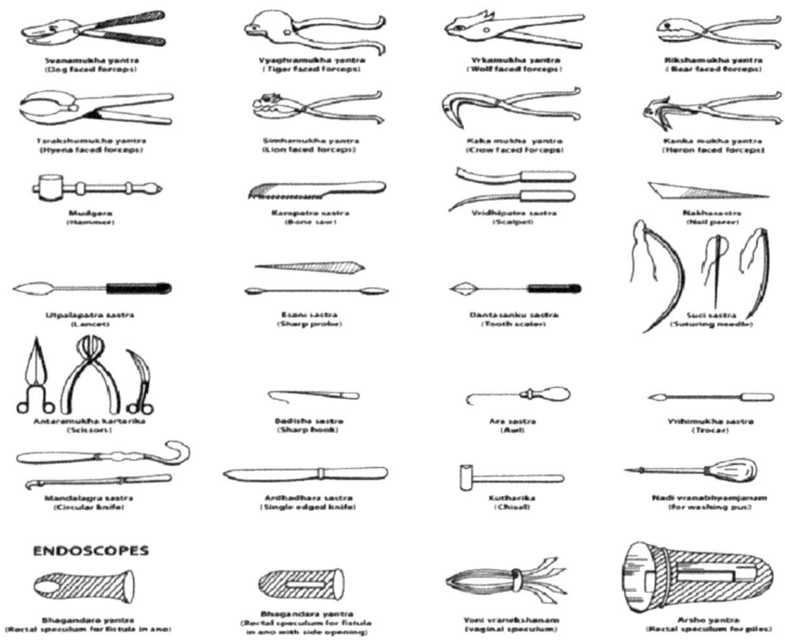
Svanamukha yantra (Dog faced forceps)
Vyaghramukha yantra (Tiger faced forceps)
Vrkamukha yantra (Wolf faced forceps)
Rikshamukha yantra (Bear faced forceps)
Tarakshumukha yantra (Hyena faced forceps)
Simhamukha yantra (Lion faced forceps)
Kaka mukha yantra (Crow faced forceps)
Kanka mukha yantra (Heron faced forceps)
Mudgara (Hammer)
Karapatra sastra (Bone saw)
Vridhipatra sastra (Scalpel)
Nakhasastra (Nail parer)
Utpalapatra sastra (Lancet)
Esani sastra (Sharp probe)
Dantasanku sastra (Tooth scaler)
Suci sastra (Suturing needle)
Antaramukha kartarika (Scissors)
Badisha sastra (Sharp hook)
Ara sastra (Awl)
Vrihimukha sastra (Trocar)
Mandalagra sastra (Circular knife)
Ardhadhara sastra (Single edged knife)
Kutharika (Chisel)
Nadi vranabhyamjanam (for washing pus)
ENDOSCOPES
Bhagandara yantra (Rectal speculum for fistula in ano)
Bhagandara yantra (Rectal speculum for fistula in ano with side opening)
Yoni vranekshanam (vaginal speculum)
Arsho yantra (Rectal speculum for piles)

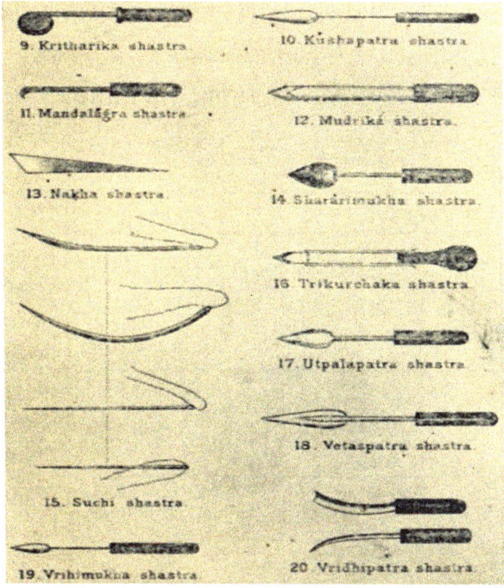
9. Kritharika shastra
10. Kushapatra shastra
11. Mandalāgra shastra
12. Mudrikā shastra
13. Nakha shastra
14. Sharārimukha shastra
16. Trikurchaka shastra
17. Utpalapatra shastra
18. Vetaspatra shastra
15. Suchi shastra
19. Vrihimukha shastra
20. Vridhipatra shastra

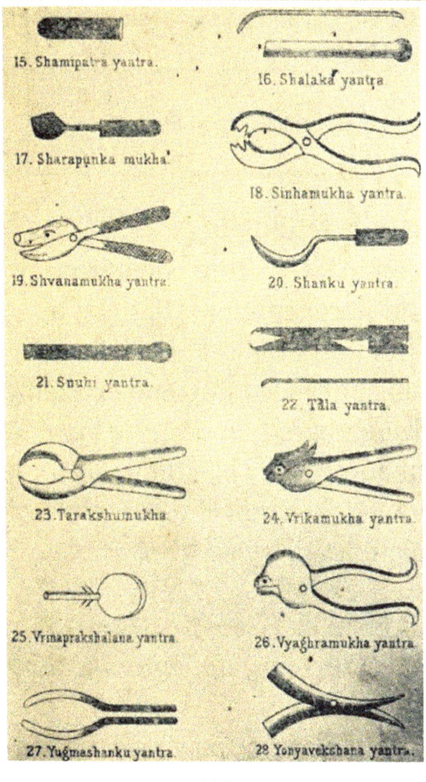
15. Shamipatra yantra.
16. Shalakā yantra
17. Sharapunka mukha
18. Sinhamukha yantra.
19. Shvanamukha yantra
20. Shanku yantra.
21. Snuhi yantra.
22. Tāla yantra.
23. Tarakshumukha
24. Vrikamukha yantra.
25. Vrinaprakshalana yantra
26. Vyaghramukha yantra
27. Yugmashanku yantra
28 Yonyavekshana yantra.

Plate 4 (turn0image7): Sharp instruments—*Kritharika* (ring knife), *Kushapatra* (bistoury), *Mandalagra*, *Mudrika*, *Nakhasastra*, *Shararimukha*, *Trikurchaka*, *Vrihimukha*, and more.

Notable Close-ups

Instrument	Description	Use
Sinhamukha/ Shvanamukha Yantras	Shaped like animal mouths (lion, dog), likely for grasping or extracting small objects	Removing bone spines or deeply embedded foreign bodies
Shanku (Trocar)	Pointed tubular instrument for drainage	Puncturing abscesses, draining fluids
Nakhasastra	Nail-knife, curved or straight, ~9 finger-width long	Excising small lesions or paring nails
Trikurchaka & Kushapatra	Multi-edged cutting tools—three-edged knife & bistoury	Draining abscesses, precise incisions
Mandalagra / Mudrika	Circular and ring-shaped blades	Excision and scraping in confined regions

Design & Ergonomic Highlights

- Crafted predominantly from steel/iron, with attention to sharpening and sterilization for optimal use.
- Many blunt Yantras mimic animal forms—lion, tiger, dog, bird—providing enhanced grip and anatomical functionality.
- Ergonomic design based on *Anguli Pramana* (approx. finger width) for comfortable handling over long procedures, aligning with modern surgical tool ergonomics.
- Stepwise depiction of *Ksharakarma*

1. Preparing the Kṣhāra (Caustic Alkali)

- Combust plant parts (e.g., *Apāmārga/Kalāmūṣka*) with lime, ash, and herbal additives.
- Filter the ash with water or cow urine (~21 passes), then boil

down to obtain a reddish, slimy paste or powder—the *Kṣāra*.

- Further processing with shells, conch, pearls, animal biles yields *Madhyama* (medium) potency *Kṣāra*, stored in iron pots until matured.

2. Bṛūhas (Pre Procedure Setup)

- Thorough patient assessment (*doṣa*, disease severity, body strength).
- Clean and anesthetize the target area (e.g., piles or granuloma), with bowel prep and antisepsis.
- Ensure sterile equipment (proctoscope, applicators, cotton swabs) are ready.

3. Applying the Kṣhāra (Kṣāra-Prayoga)

- Expose the lesion with a speculum or proctoscope.
- Use a heated iron rod or sterile applicator to deposit a thin layer of *Kṣāra* on the lesion surface and surrounding margins.
- Wait for the defined period (measured in "*matras*"); tissues begin coagulating and crusting.
- Protect adjacent healthy tissue with soaked cotton swabs.

4. Cleaning & Cooling

- Remove the dried *Kṣāra* with moist cotton swabs.
- Apply a soothing mixture of honey + ghee, followed by milk or gruels, and finalize with cool oil or herbal pastes to promote healing.

5. Post Procedure Care & Follow-up

- Dressing is changed daily; healing progresses from scab formation to sloughing and healthy tissue growth by ~7–10 days .
- Full healing typically occurs within 3–4 weeks with minimal scarring. Studies report no recurrence at 21 days in piles—often extending to months of follow-up .

Visual Healing Timeline (Based on Clinical Images)

- Image 1: Pre op—inflamed lesion or granuloma.
- Image 2: During *Kṣārakarma*—paste applied, visible whitening/coagulation.
- Image 3: Day 1–5 Post op—scabbing begins; early granulation tissue visible.
- Image 4: Day 7 onward—slough resolved; healthy tissue; full healing by ~1 month.

Key Benefits & Considerations

- Chemical cauterization avoids surgical cutting—leading to less bleeding, faster recovery, and lower recurrence.
- Potency tailored to tissue: *Mṛdu* (mild), *Madhyama* (moderate), *Tīkṣṇa* (strong) based on lesion depth.
- Effectively used for piles, fistula, granulomas, *nasa*l polyps, keloids, cervical erosion, etc.
- Post-care includes anti-inflammatory diet and supportive herbal dressings (e.g., sesame-ghee paste).

In Summary

Kṣhārakarma is a meticulous, multi stage Ayurvedic parasurgical technique using plant-derived *alkali* to chemically excise unhealthy tissue. When performed correctly, it offers a controlled, minimally invasive approach with effective healing and low recurrence—demonstrating profound sophistication in ancient medical science.

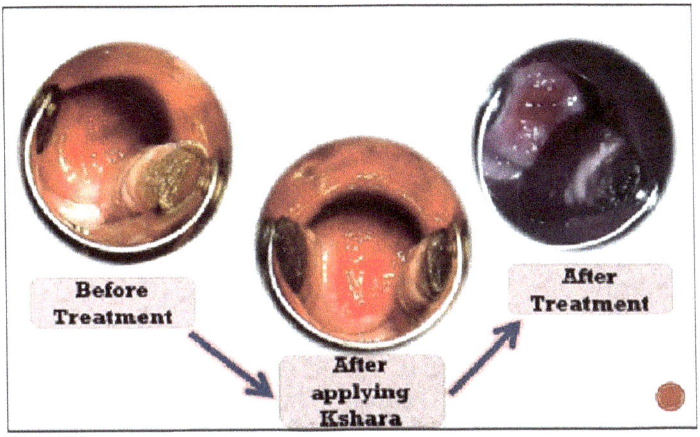
Before Treatment
After applying Kshara
After Treatment

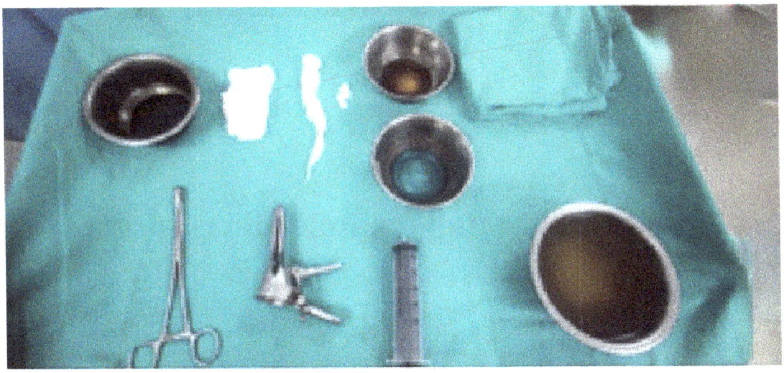

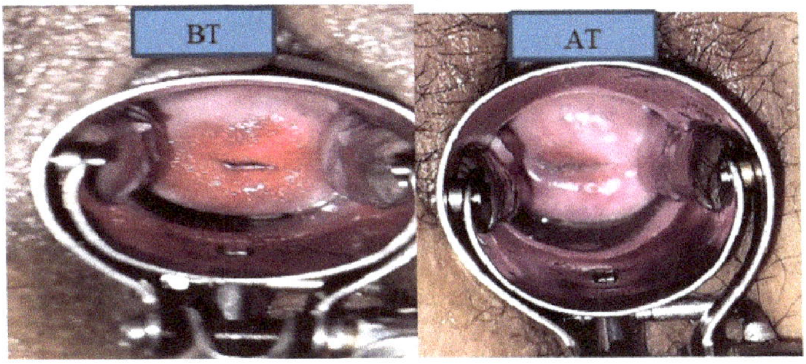
BT
AT

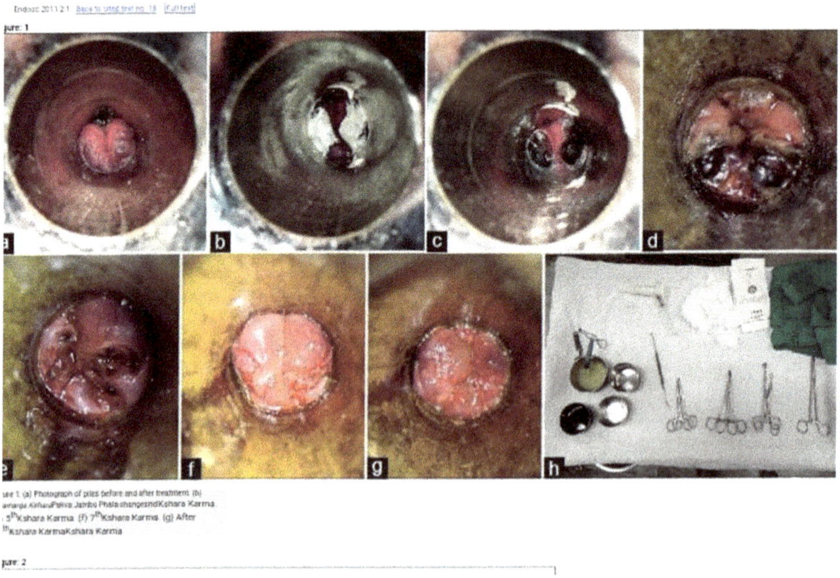

Modern laser setup (console, fibers, probes)

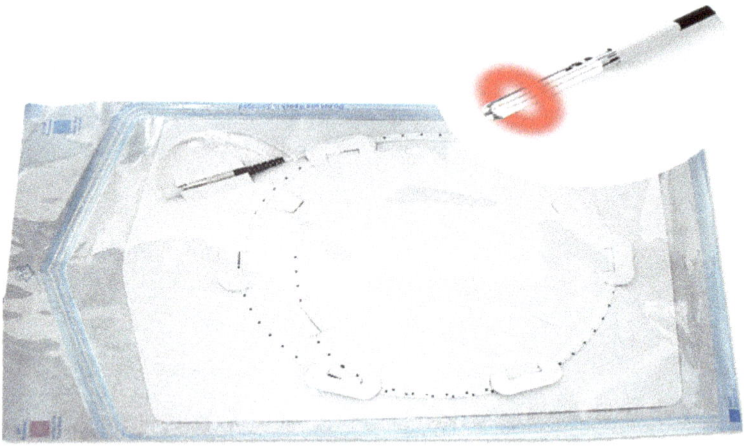

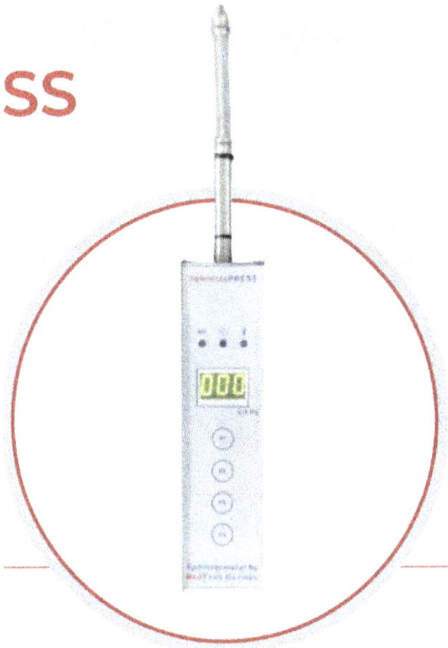
SS

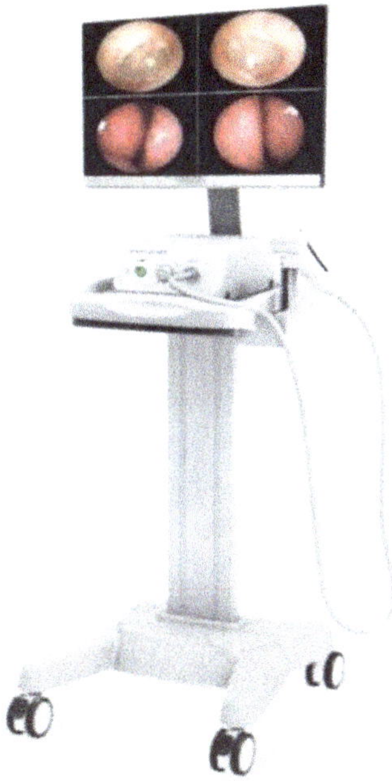

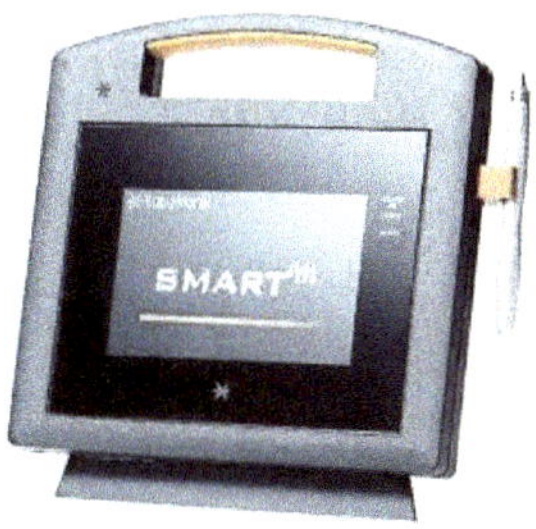
SMART

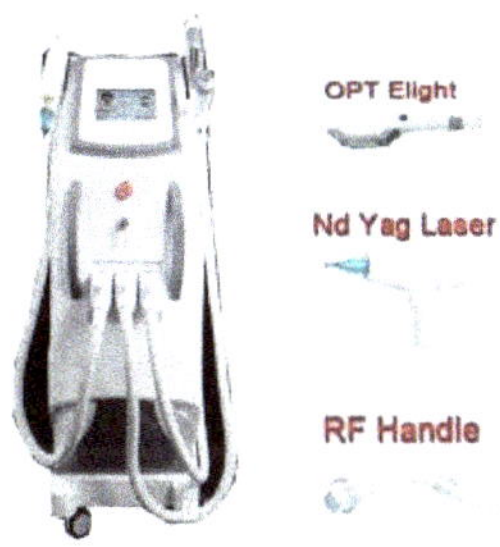
OPT Elight
Nd Yag Laser
RF Handle

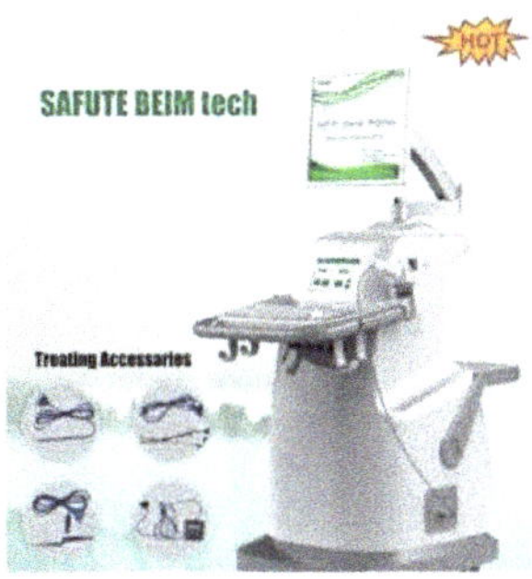
HOT
SAFUTE BEIM tech
Treating Accessories

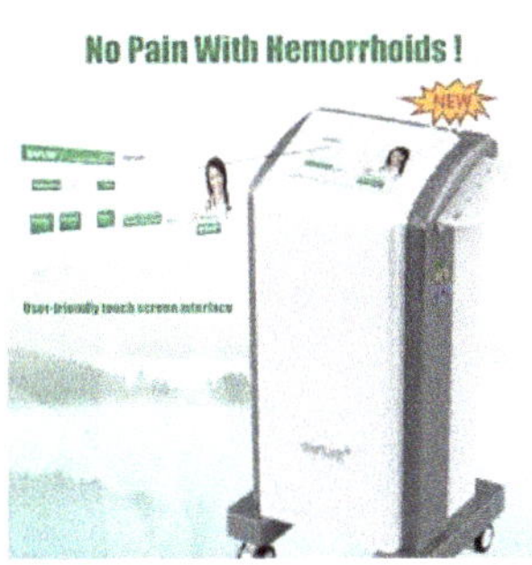
No Pain With Hemorrhoids !
NEW

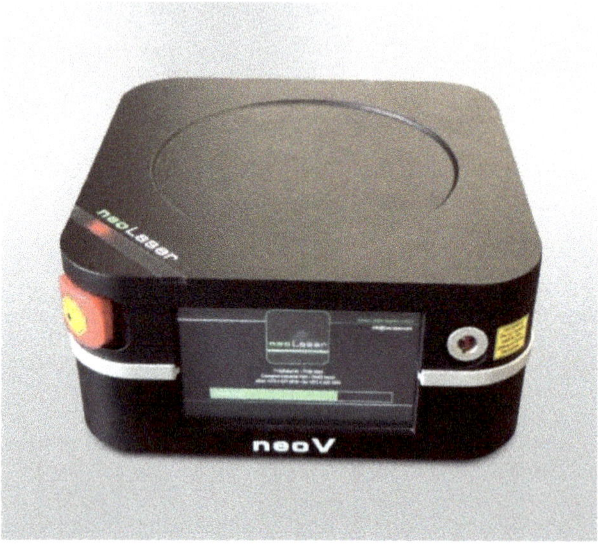

Integrated OT table layout with dual instrument trays

References

1. Sharma PV. Sushruta Samhita with Commentary by Dalhana
2. Gokhale A., (2019). Modern Integration of Ksharasutra in Colorectal Surgery
3. Sahave P., (2024). Laser and Ayurveda in Anal Surgery: Case Reports and Techniques
4. Indian Proctology Association Guidelines (2023 Edition)

Ch. 23
Training Modern Surgeons in Ayurvedic Philosophy

"A skilled hand heals the body, but an awakened mind heals the whole being."

Modern surgeons are highly trained in anatomy, pathology, and precision techniques — but in an age of integrative medicine, there is a growing realization that healing is not merely technical, it is holistic. This chapter explores how the timeless philosophies of Ayurveda can enrich the training of today's surgical practitioners, transforming them from mechanical operators into healers who align with nature, ethics, and individualized care.

1. Why Philosophical Training Matters

In Ayurveda, the Vaidya (physician) is expected to possess:

- *Buddhi* (clinical intelligence),
- *Shraddha* (faith and compassion),
- *Desha-Kala-Jnana* (knowledge of patient's geography, season, and environment) and above all, *Atmabala* (personal integrity and self-discipline).

Training modern surgeons in Ayurvedic philosophy helps to:

- Encourage empathetic car
- Enhance diagnostic depth using *Tridosha* theory
- Promote preventive and lifestyle-oriented post-surgical strategies
- Restore the concept of the surgeon as a healer, not merely a technician

2. Foundational Philosophies to Teach

Concept	Meaning	Surgical Application
TriDosha (Vata, Pitta, Kapha)	Biological energies	Guides patient constitution and healing potential
Prakriti	Individual constitution	Influences anesthesia response, recovery time
Srotas	Bodily channels	Understanding fistula tracts, wound drainage
Dhatu & Mala	Tissues & waste	Tissue regeneration and wound discharge management
Ojas	Vital energy	Correlates with immune strength post-surgery
Satva, Rajas, Tamas	Mental states	Understanding stress impact on surgical recovery

3. Suggested Curriculum for Surgical Students

A short-term module or certificate course in Ayurvedic philosophy for surgeons may include:

Module 1: Philosophy & Ethics

- Role of the *Vaidya* as a healer
- The *Dhanvantari* Oath (Ayurvedic version of Hippocratic Oath)
- Ethical decision-making through Ayurvedic lens

Module 2: Ayurvedic Anatomy & Physiology

- *Srotas* and *Dhatu* system
- *Tridosha* physiology in disease and recovery

Module 3: Practical Ayurveda for Surgeons

- Pre- and post-operative dietetics (*Pathya-APathya*)
- *Panchakarma* and *Rasayana* in surgical preparation and recovery
- Herbal asepsis and medicated dressings

Module 4: Integrative Clinical Decision-Making

- Case studies of Ayurvedic + modern surgical integration
- *Tridosha*-based preoperative planning
- Incorporating *Shalya Tantra* tools when relevant

4. Case Study: A Surgeon Transformed

Dr. Neeraj, a colorectal surgeon trained in laser proctology, enrolled in a 6-month Ayurvedic philosophy course.

Outcomes:

- Improved rapport with patients through deeper constitutional assessment
- Adopted *Triphalā ghṛita* and *Ashwagandha* in post-op care
- Noticed fewer complications and higher patient satisfaction scores
- Now delivers lectures on "*Tridosha* and Recovery Physiology" in surgical forums

5. The Inner Discipline of a Surgeon

Ayurveda emphasizes *Swasthya* (personal health) of the physician.

Recommendations for surgeon wellness:

- Daily *Dinacharya*: Wake early, *Pranayama*, and mild *Abhyanga* (oil self-massage)
- Sattvic diet to maintain mental clarity
- Meditative grounding before surgeries to enhance presence and compassion

These practices help reduce burnout, improve decision-making, and align the practitioner with Ayurveda's central idea: "*Yat Pinde Tat Brahmande*" — the microcosm reflects the macrocosm.

6. Tools for Training Integration

- E-learning modules with animated concepts of *Dosha/Dhatu*

- Interactive diagnostic simulations for surgical Ayurveda application
- Internships at integrative centers like AVP, KLE Ayurveda, or Banaras Ayurveda
- Joint CME programs with AYUSH and surgical institutions

7. Image Ideas

Modern Surgical Curriculum vs Ayurvedic Enrichment Points

Category	**Modern Surgical Curriculum**	**Ayurvedic Enrichment Points**
Philosophy & Foundation	Evidence-based, anatomy/ physiology centered	*TriDosha* (*Vata, Pitta, Kapha*), Srotas (channels), *Prakriti*-based personalization
Anatomy & Physiology	Detailed cadaveric dissection, imaging-guided understanding	*Marma* points (vital points), concept of *Dhatu*s, understanding body through energy centers
Surgical Techniques	Open, laparoscopic, robotic surgeries	Ancient techniques like *Ksharasutra* for fistula, *Agnikarma* for cauterization
Instrumentation	Stainless steel, high-tech tools, robotic systems	Herbal pastes, hand-crafted tools (ancient), natural cauterizing agents like alkaline threads
Infection Control	Aseptic technique, antibiotics, sterilization	Use of antimicrobial herbs (*Neem*, Turmeric), wound cleansing with medicated decoctions
Pain Management	Opioids, NSAIDs, anesthesia	*Taila abhyanga* (oil massage), *Shirodhara*, herbal analgesics, mind-body balance
Post-operative Care	ICU monitoring, physiotherapy, biochemical follow-up	*Rasayana* (rejuvenation therapy), *Panchakarma* detoxification, diet-tailored healing

Surgical Ethics & Training	Modern codes (Hippocratic, informed consent, patient autonomy)	Ethical conduct in *Sushruta Samhita*, *Guru-Shishya* parampara, moral obligations of the Vaidya
Diagnostic Principles	Imaging (MRI, CT, USG), histopathology, labs	*Nadi Pariksha* (pulse diagnosis), *Drik-Vikriti* (observation), *Dosha* imbalance analysis
Holistic Integration	Generally systems-specific, less holistic unless integrated medicine is taught	Treats root cause through body–mind–spirit alignment, lifestyle corrections, and *Satvavajaya Chikitsa*
Education & Skill Development	Simulations, OSCE, cadaver labs, structured residency	Observation, gradual hands-on exposure, Shravan (listening) → *Manan* (reflection) → *Nididhyasan*

Diagram: Tridosha influence on surgical recovery

- Quote graphics from *Sushruta*, *Charaka*, and modern integrative pioneers
- Photos of Ayurvedic surgical training centers and integrative workshops

---

References

1. Sushruta Samhita – Shalya Tantra chapters
2. Tripathi B. (2020). Ayurvedic Principles for Modern Physicians
3. AIIMS Delhi & CCRAS Collaborative Module: Ayurveda for Medical Graduates

International Laser Proctology Training Program

By Dr. Praveen Sahave

MS (Gen. Surg.), FRHS, FICS, FRACS (Proctology)

Founder of Abhyudaya Laser Proctology Institute, Nagpur

Course Title:
"Integrative Laser Proctology: Bridging Ayurvedic Principles & Surgical Precision"

Location Options:

- Abhyudaya Piles Laser Hospital, Nagpur (India)
- Global Partner Centers (Dubai, Colombo, Kuala Lumpur)
- Hybrid Format: Live Online + Hands-On Offline

Duration:

7-Day Intensive Training

- Pre-Course Online Module Access (1 Week Prior)
- Post-Course Support (1 Month, Virtual)

Who Can Attend?

- BAMS / MS *Shalya Tantra* Practitioners
- MS General Surgery / Colorectal Surgeons
- Laser Specialists / Proctologists
- Integrative Medicine Doctors

Key Learning Objectives:

- Master minimally invasive laser procedures (LHP, FILAC, fissurectomy)
- Integrate Ayurvedic therapies (*Panchakarma*, *Rasayana*) for better outcomes

- Understand *Dosha*-based surgical planning
- Learn post-op wound healing using Ayurvedic oils, diet & leech therapy
- Acquire hands-on experience with laser machines and simulators

Topics Covered (Modules):

1. Fundamentals of Laser Physics & Safety
2. Laser Hemorrhoidoplasty (LHP)
3. Laser Fissurectomy & Anal Tags
4. Fistula-in-Ano Closure (FILAC) Techniques
5. Pilonidal Sinus Management
6. Hybrid Approach: Laser + Ksharsutra
7. Ayurvedic Pre & Post-op Protocols
8. Managing Complications & Ethics
9. Global Certification & Medical Legal Aspects

Hands-On Procedures Include:

- Simulation models for laser use
- OT observation of live cases (where available)
- Handling BIEM, Diode, and CO_2 Laser machines

Certification:

Internationally Recognized Certificate in Laser Proctology

- CPD/CME Points (Where Applicable)
- Alumni Access to Global Forum

Trainer Profile: Dr. Praveen Sahave

- Over 15 years of surgical experience
- 5,000+ free surgeries for underserved patients
- Brand Ambassador of BIEM Laser Tech (China)
- Awarded: Times Healthcare Achiever, Sakal Excellence, FRACS (Proctology)
- Founder: Abhyudaya Piles Laser Hospital – Rs. 2 Cr+ annual

turnover
- 170K+ followers on Instagram promoting proctology awareness

Course Fees:
- Rs. 50,000 – Rs.75,000 INR (India)
- $750 – $1,000 USD (International)
- Includes: course materials, simulator access, certification
- Accommodation packages optional

How to Register:
- Email: pppsahave@gmial.com
- Website: www.pilesfistulacure.com
- WhatsApp: +91- 99707 43318
- Instagram: @drpraveensahave

Bonus:
- Lifetime mentor support
- Free consultation templates
- Legal consent formats
- Digital *Dosha*-surgical planner toolkit

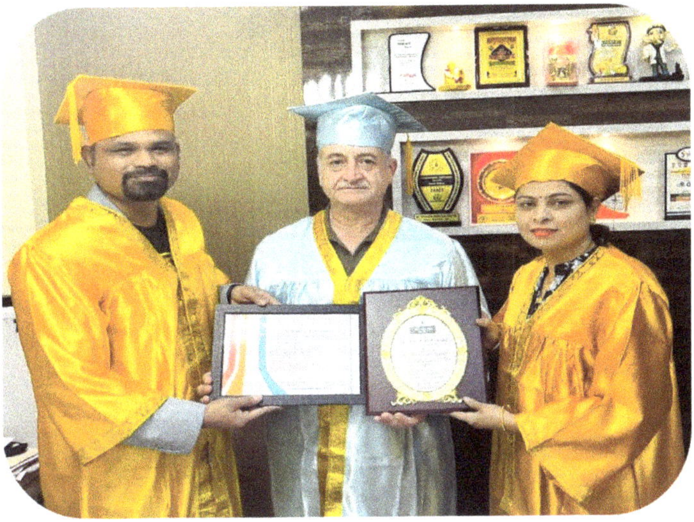

Dr. Firoj Sir MBBS MS (Laparoscopic Surgeon) from Jordon Joinded our Advance Laser and Ayurveda Ksharsutra Course

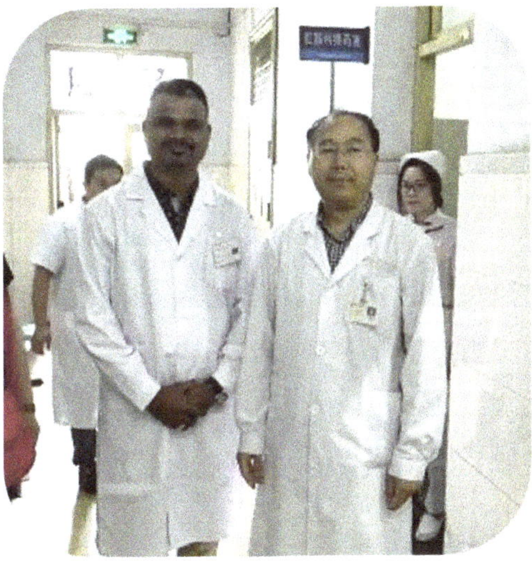

Dr. Shie From Zhengzhaou China Trained Dr. Praveen Sahave

Live Laser Proctology Workshop

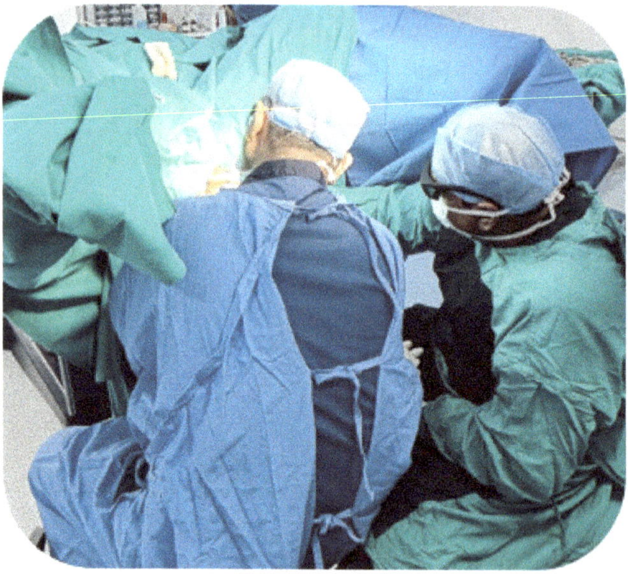

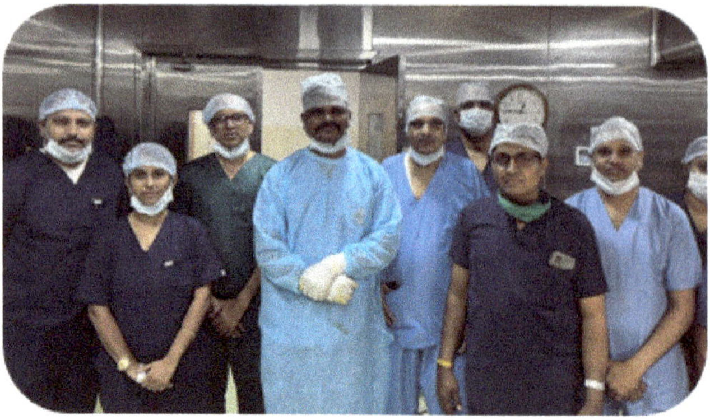

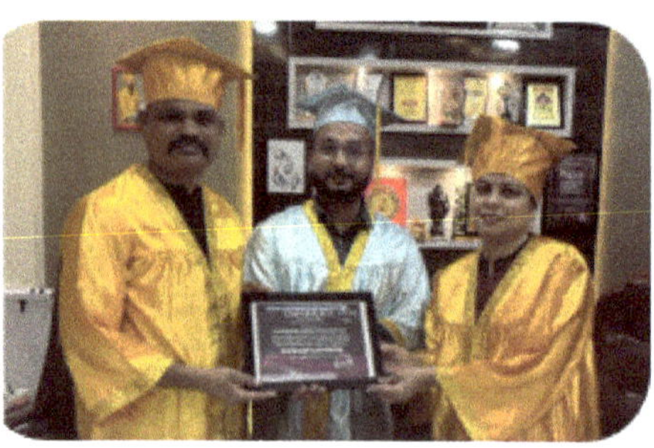

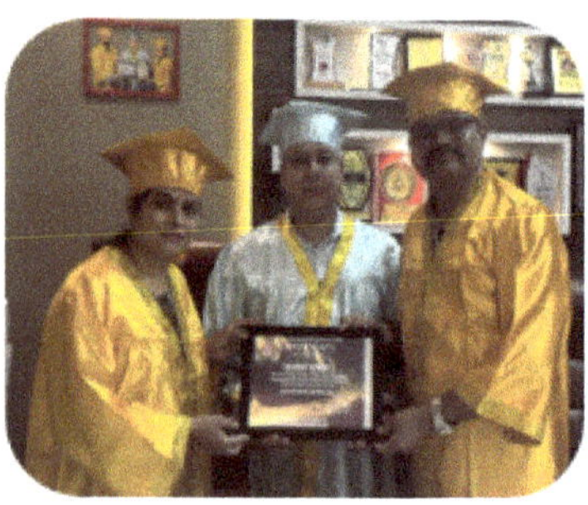

Laser Training Doctor From All Over India

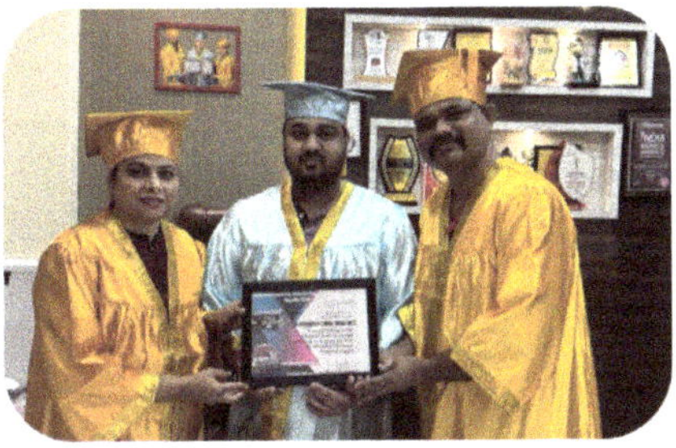

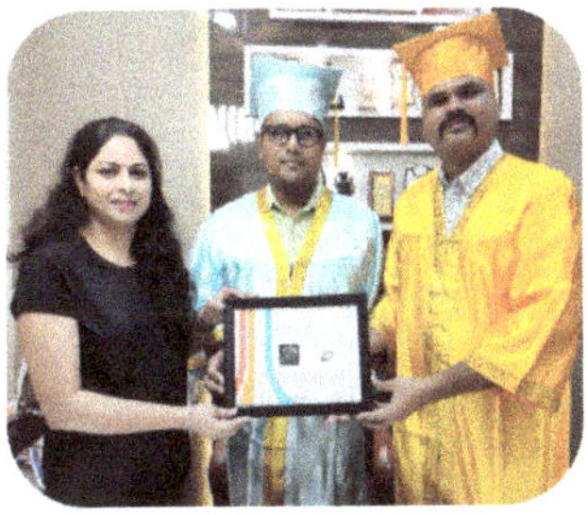

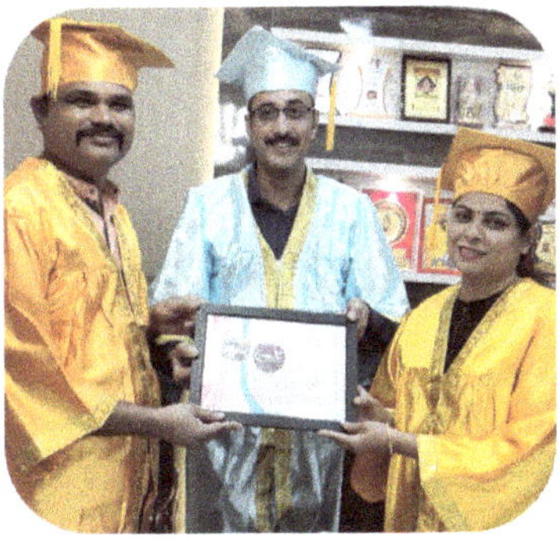

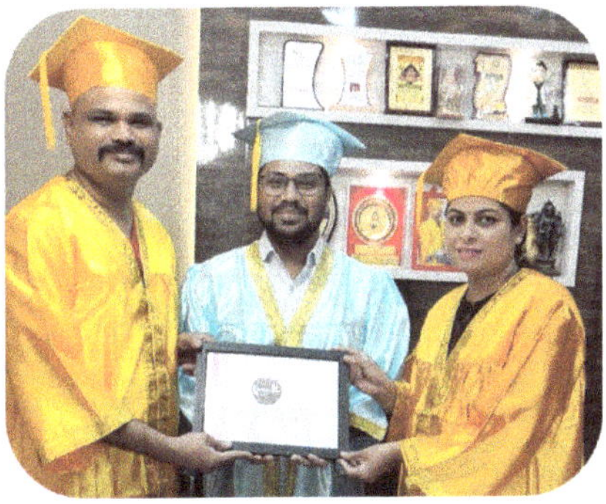

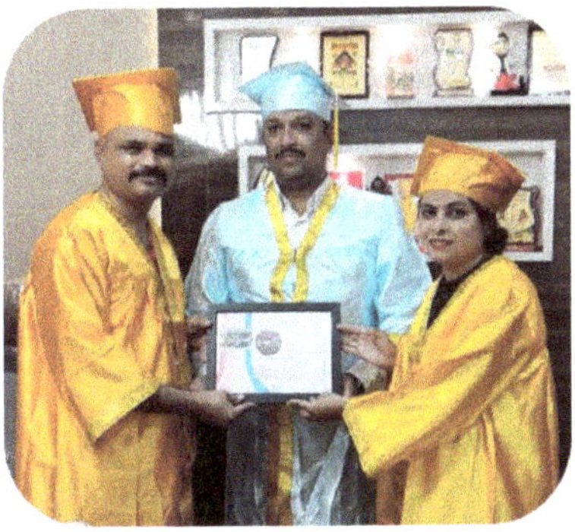

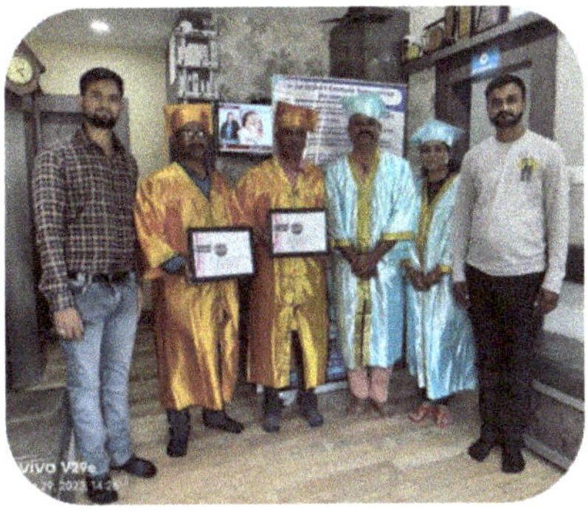

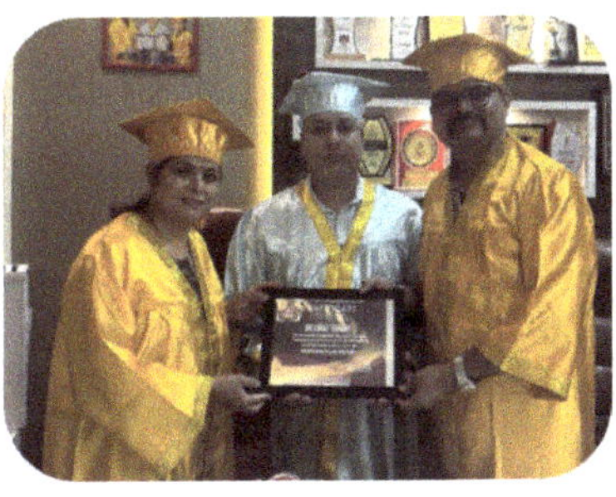

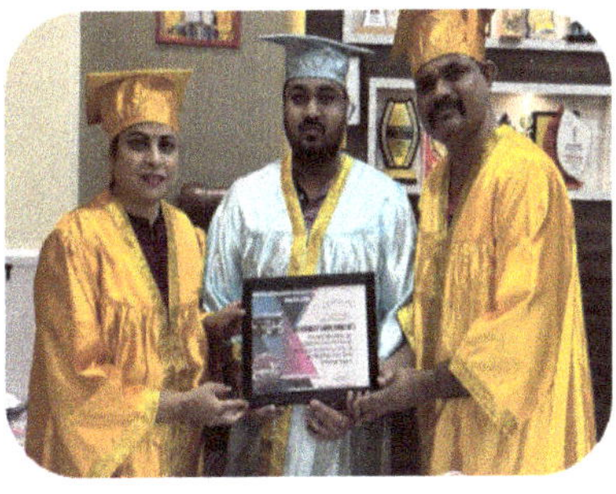

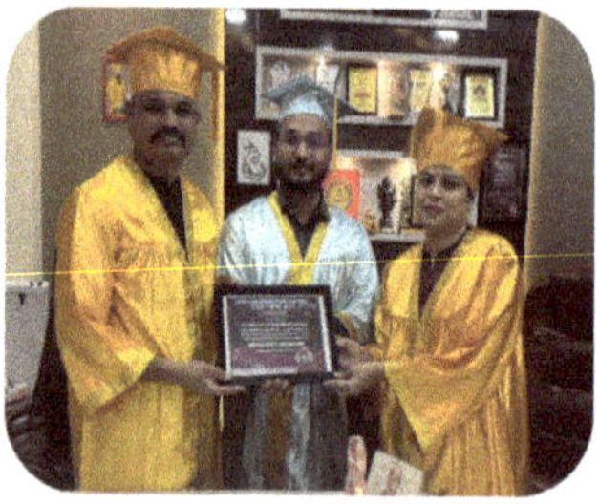
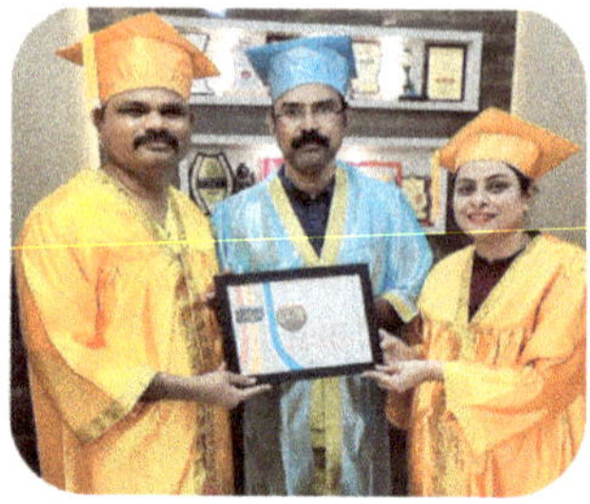
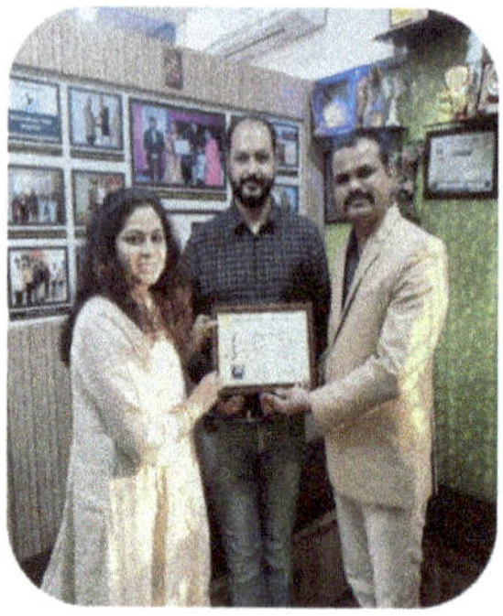
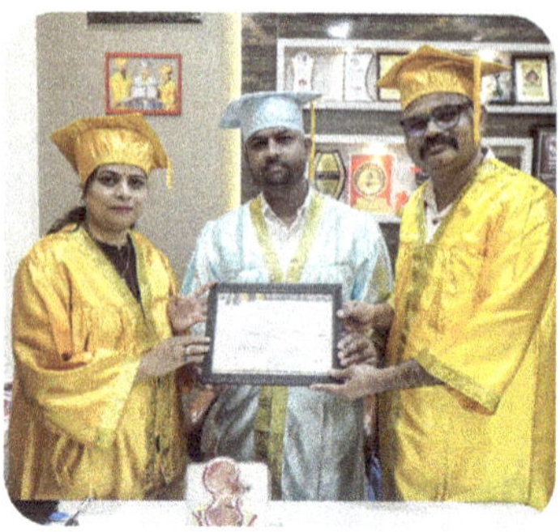
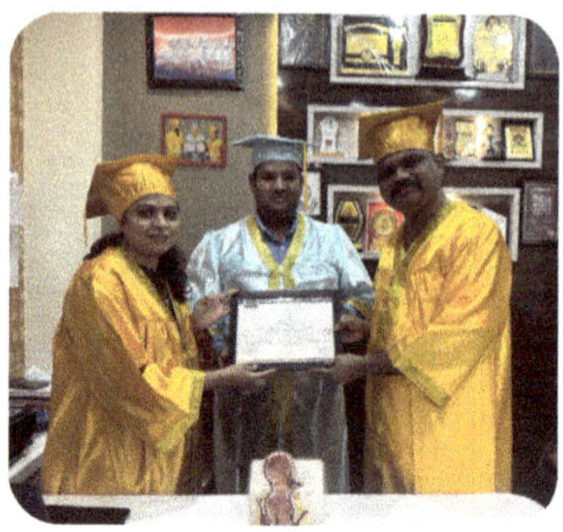
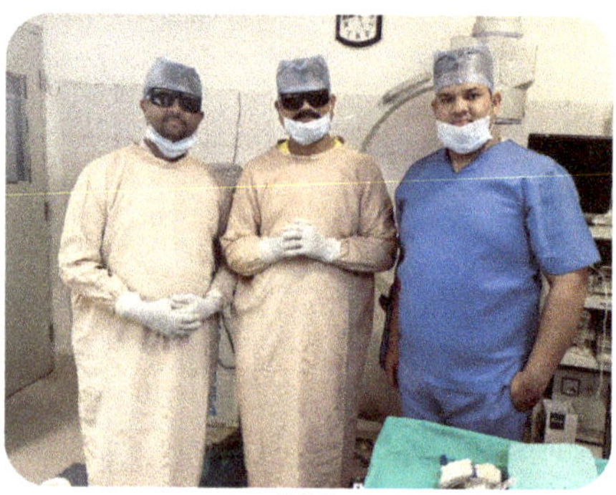

International Laser Training of Dr. Praveen Sahave at Zhengzhou China

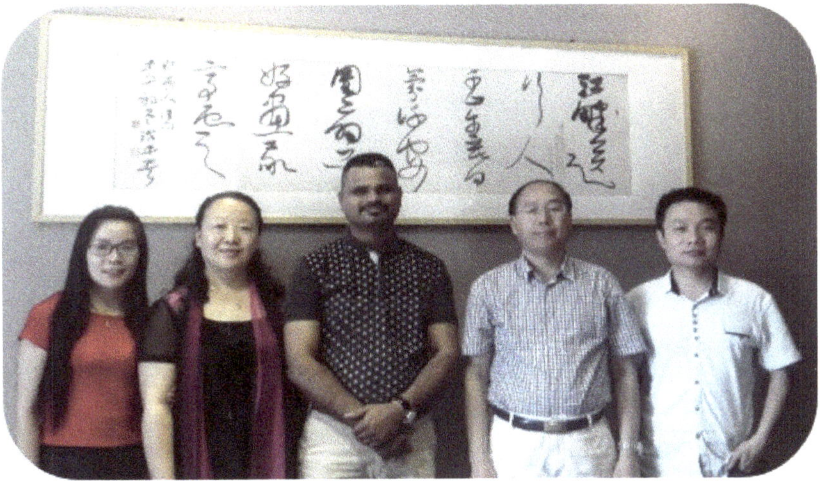

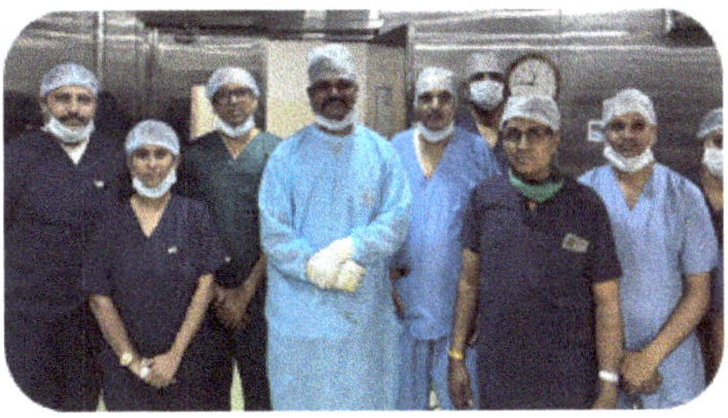

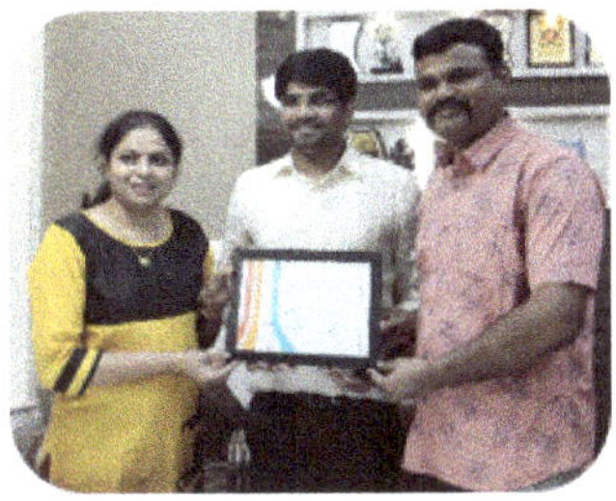

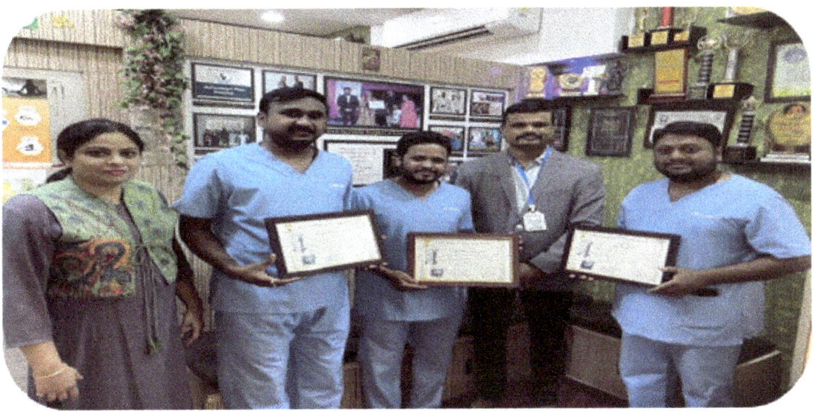

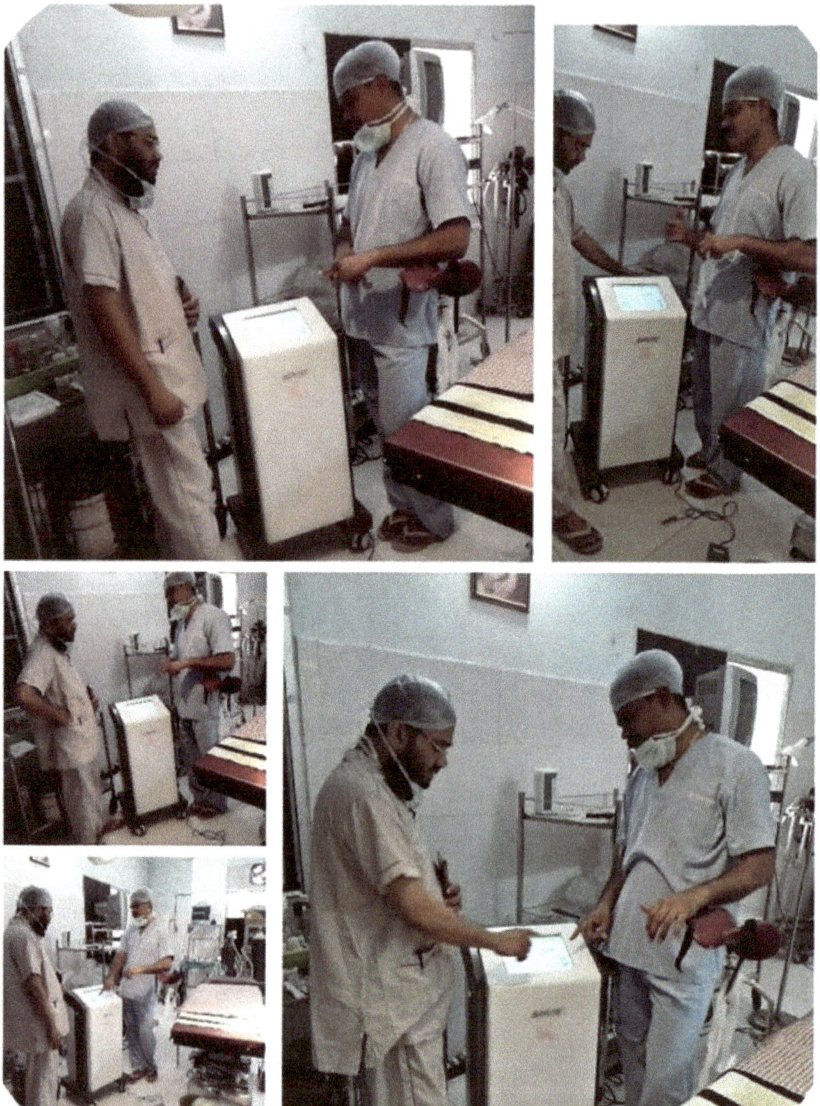

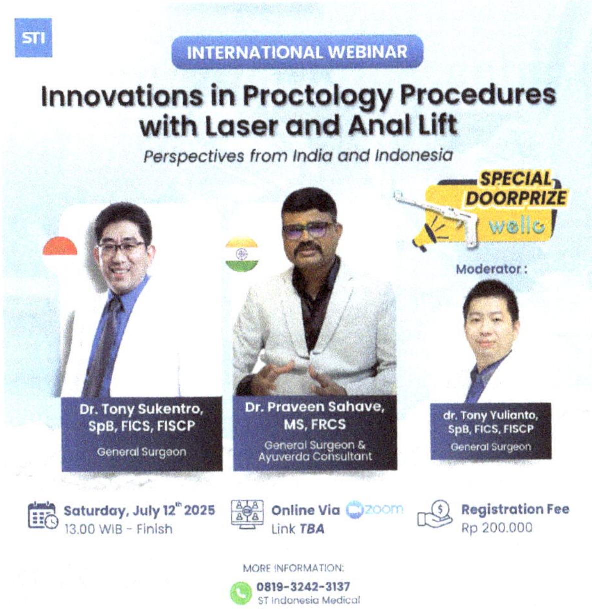
STI
INTERNATIONAL WEBINAR
Innovations in Proctology Procedures with Laser and Anal Lift
Perspectives from India and Indonesia
SPECIAL DOORPRIZE
wello
Moderator :
Dr. Tony Sukentro, SpB, FICS, FISCP
General Surgeon
Dr. Praveen Sahave, MS, FRCS
General Surgeon & Ayuverda Consultant
dr. Tony Yulianto, SpB, FICS, FISCP
General Surgeon
Saturday, July 12th 2025
13.00 WIB - Finish
Online Via zoom
Link TBA
Registration Fee
Rp 200.000
MORE INFORMATION:
0819-3242-3137
ST Indonesia Medical

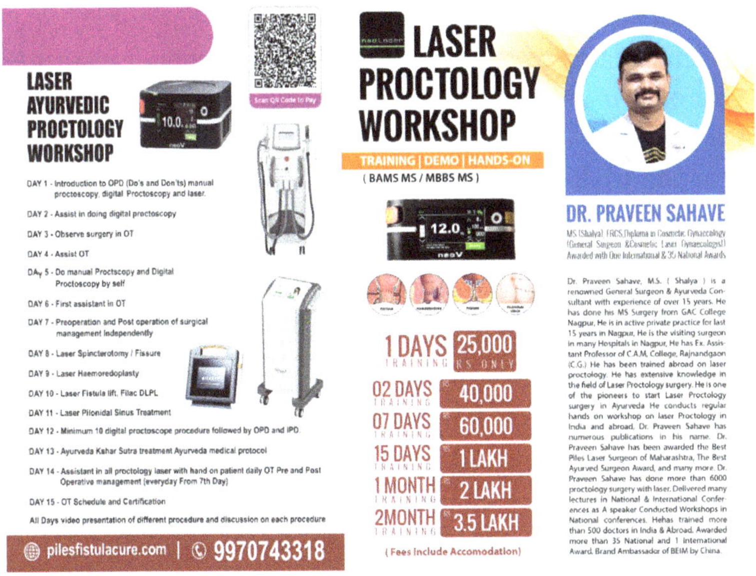
LASER AYURVEDIC PROCTOLOGY WORKSHOP
Scan QR Code to Pay
DAY 1 - Introduction to OPD (Do's and Don'ts) manual proctoscopy, digital Proctoscopy and laser.
DAY 2 - Assist in doing digital proctoscopy
DAY 3 - Observe surgery in OT
DAY 4 - Assist OT
DAy 5 - Do manual Proctscopy and Digital Proctoscopy by self
DAY 6 - First assistant in OT
DAY 7 - Preoperation and Post operation of surgical management Independently
DAY 8 - Laser Spincterotomy / Fissure
DAY 9 - Laser Haemoredoplasty
DAY 10 - Laser Fistula lift, Filac DLPL
DAY 11 - Laser Pilonidal Sinus Treatment
DAY 12 - Minimum 10 digital proctoscope procedure followed by OPD and IPD.
DAY 13 - Ayurveda Kahar Sutra treatment Ayurveda medical protocol
DAY 14 - Assistant in all proctology laser with hand on patient daily OT Pre and Post Operative management (everyday From 7th Day)
DAY 15 - OT Schedule and Certification
All Days video presentation of different procedure and discussion on each procedure
pilesfistulacure.com | 9970743318
LASER PROCTOLOGY WORKSHOP
TRAINING | DEMO | HANDS-ON
(BAMS MS / MBBS MS)
1 DAYS TRAINING 25,000 RS ONLY
02 DAYS TRAINING 40,000
07 DAYS TRAINING 60,000
15 DAYS TRAINING 1 LAKH
1 MONTH TRAINING 2 LAKH
2MONTH TRAINING 3.5 LAKH
(Fees Include Accomodation)
DR. PRAVEEN SAHAVE
MS (Shalya) FRCS Diploma in Cosmetic Gynaecology (General Surgeon &Cosmetic Laser Gynaecologist) Awarded with One International & 35 National Awards
Dr. Praveen Sahave, M.S. (Shalya) is a renowned General Surgeon & Ayurveda Consultant with experience of over 15 years. He has done his MS Surgery from GAC College Nagpur, He is in active private practice for last 15 years in Nagpur, He is the visiting surgeon in many Hospitals in Nagpur, He has Ex. Assistant Professor of C.A.M. College, Rajnandgaon (C.G.) He has been trained abroad on laser proctology. He has extensive knowledge in the field of Laser Proctology surgery. He is one of the pioneers to start Laser Proctology surgery in Ayurveda He conducts regular hands on workshop on laser Proctology in India and abroad. Dr. Praveen Sahave has numerous publications in his name. Dr. Praveen Sahave has been awarded the Best Piles Laser Surgeon of Maharashtra, The Best Ayurved Surgeon Award, and many more. Dr. Praveen Sahave has done more than 6000 proctology surgery with laser. Delivered many lectures in National & International Conferences as A speaker Conducted Workshops in National conferences. Hehas trained more than 500 doctors in India & Abroad. Awarded more than 35 National and 1 International Award. Brand Ambassador of BEIM by China.

Ch. 24
Sterilization, Suturing & Dressing: Best of Both Worlds

"Merging the purity of tradition with the precision of modern science ensures wounds heal both safely and swiftly."

In surgical practice, infection control, wound closure, and dressing techniques are paramount to ensure successful outcomes. Ayurveda and modern surgery offer unique insights and tools in these domains. This chapter discusses how the best practices from both systems can be synergized, optimizing patient recovery with minimal complications.

1. Sterilization: Ancient Practices & Modern Standards

Ayurvedic Sterilization Insights:

- Traditional *Sushruta Samhita* describes the use of heat (*Agni*) and medicated decoctions (*Kwatha*) for cleaning instruments.
- Use of *Triphala Kwatha* and *Neem* decoctions for antiseptic washing.
- Practice of Sun-drying (*Aditya Shakti*) for instruments and linens to harness natural UV rays.
- Smoke fumigation with herbs like *Nagkesar* and *Chandan* for air purification.

Modern Sterilization Techniques:

- Autoclaving (steam sterilization at 121°C under pressure)
- Chemical sterilants (Glutaraldehyde, Ethylene oxide)
- Use of sterile disposables for reducing cross-infection
- UV sterilizers and HEPA filtration in OT air systems

Integrative Approach:

- Pre-sterilization soaking of instruments in herbal antiseptics (e.g., *Neem*, *Tulsi*)
- Use of herbal fumigation alongside standard sterilization to reduce microbial load in the OT
- Awareness of Ayurveda's emphasis on Sattvic environment — clean, calm, and purified

2. Suturing: Materials and Techniques

Ayurvedic Surgical Suturing:

- Suturing materials described included Silk threads, Cotton threads, and natural fibers coated with herbal pastes.
- *Sushruta* mentions *Kshaara* (alkaline substances) applied to sutures for antiseptic purposes.
- Knotting techniques focused on secure closure without tissue strangulation.
- Use of Leech therapy for venous congestion post-suturing.

Modern Suturing Techniques:

- Variety of absorbable (Vicryl, Catgut) and non-absorbable (Nylon, Prolene) sutures
- Advanced needle designs for minimal trauma
- Staples and surgical adhesives as alternatives
- Microsurgical suturing for delicate structures

Combined Insights:

- Herbal coating on sutures (e.g., Turmeric, *Neem* extracts) can reduce infection and inflammation.
- Selection of suture type based on *Dosha* and tissue type (e.g., *Kapha* dominant patients may benefit from faster absorbable materials due to slower healing).
- Complement suturing with *Rasayana* herbs to enhance tissue repair.

3. Dressing: Traditional Medicinal Dressings & Modern Advances

Ayurvedic Wound Dressings:

- Use of *Jatyadi Taila* and *Ghrita*: Known for antimicrobial and healing properties.
- Herbal powders (*Churna*) like *Yashad Bhasma*, *Haridra* (Turmeric), and *Guggulu* applied directly.
- Application of Medicated Ghee and Oils to maintain moist wound healing.
- Dressings made from Cotton, flax, or silk soaked in medicinal decoctions.

Modern Wound Dressings

- Sterile gauze, hydrogels, alginate dressing.
- Antimicrobial dressings impregnated with silver or honey
- Vacuum-assisted closure (VAC) for chronic wounds
- Use of synthetic semi-permeable films to maintain ideal moisture *Bala*nce

Best Practices Integration:

- Combine herbal medicated oils with sterile modern dressings to maintain asepsis and enhance healing.
- Use natural anti-inflammatory agents such as turmeric-infused dressings.
- Monitor wound microenvironment with modern devices but apply Ayurvedic formulations for *Bala*nced healing.

4. Infection Control: Dual System Strategies

- Ayurveda emphasizes maintaining *Ojas* (vital energy) to resist infection; thus, patient immunity is enhanced alongside mechanical asepsis.
- Use of herbal antiseptics as adjuncts reduces antibiotic resistance risks.
- Integration of modern antibiotic stewardship with Ayurvedic

immune-modulators (e.g., *Guduchi*, *Ashwagandha*).

5. Illustrations and Tables (For Word/Print Format)

- Stepwise diagrams of herbal instrument sterilization vs autoclaving
- Comparative table: Ayurvedic vs Modern suture materials and healing outcomes
- Photographs of *Jatyadi Taila* application and modern dressing techniques
- Flowchart: Integrative wound management protocol

References

1. Sushruta Samhita – Shalya Tantra (Sterilization & Suturing)
2. Tripathi B. (2018). Ayurvedic Wound Management
3. WHO Guidelines on Sterilization and Infection Control (2022)
4. Kumar P., Sahave P. (2023). Integrative Dressing Techniques in Proctology
5. CCRAS Reports on Medicated Dressings (2021)

Ch. 25
Ethics, Regulation and Medical Acceptance

"Integrity in innovation ensures trust and longevity in the healing arts."

Integrating Ayurveda and advanced laser proctology brings transformative potential, but it also raises important ethical questions, regulatory challenges, and questions about acceptance in the broader medical community. This chapter explores how to navigate these complex terrains responsibly, ensuring patient safety, professional credibility, and widespread adoption of integrative surgical practices.

1. Ethical Foundations in Integrative Surgery

Core Ethical Principles:

- Beneficence: Ensuring the patient's welfare by combining best treatments from both traditions.
- Non-maleficence: Avoiding harm by careful selection of therapies and technologies.
- Autonomy: Respecting patients' rights to informed choice regarding Ayurvedic and modern laser options.
- Justice: Providing equitable access to integrative care irrespective of socioeconomic status.

Ayurvedic Ethics:

- Emphasizes *Dharma* (duty) and *Satya* (truthfulness) in physician conduct
- Surgeon's role as a *Sevak* (servant) to the patient and nature.
- Maintenance of *Atmabala* (self-discipline) and ongoing

personal development.

Modern Ethical Standards:

- Adherence to institutional review boards (IRBs)
- Compliance with informed consent protocols
- Maintenance of patient confidentiality and data security

2. Regulatory Landscape

Current Status:

- Ayurveda is governed by the Central Council of Indian Medicine (CCIM) and Ministry of AYUSH.
- Surgical lasers and devices are regulated by bodies such as the FDA (US), CDSCO (India), and EMA (Europe).
- Lack of standardized guidelines for combined Ayurvedic and laser surgical protocols creates a grey zone.

Challenges:

- Integrating two distinct regulatory frameworks.
- Ensuring quality control for Ayurvedic herbal products used perioperatively.
- Monitoring adverse events and establishing reporting systems.

Proposed Solutions:

- Development of integrative guidelines jointly authored by AYUSH and surgical regulatory authorities.
- Encouraging clinical trials and evidence-based research on combined therapies.
- Establishing certification programs for surgeons practicing integrative approaches.

3. Medical Acceptance and Collaboration

Bridging the Divide:

- Historically, Ayurveda and modern surgery have operated in silos.

- Successful integrative models require mutual respect, open dialogue, and shared learning.
- Formation of interdisciplinary teams involving Ayurvedic practitioners, surgeons, and researchers.

Advocacy for Integrative Surgery:

- Presentations at surgical conferences showcasing case studies and outcomes.
- Publications in peer-reviewed international journals to build scientific credibility.
- Patient education on the benefits and limitations of integrative approaches.

4. Patient Safety and Quality Assurance

- Rigorous preoperative screening incorporating Ayurvedic and allopathic diagnostics.
- Continuous monitoring of laser device safety and performance.
- Use of standard operating procedures (SOPs) combining best practices from both fields.
- Transparent disclosure of treatment plans and expected outcomes to patients.

5. Global Trends and Future Outlook

- WHO and NIH recognize the importance of Traditional and Complementary Medicine (T&CM).
- Increasing international collaborations for research and regulation harmonization.
- Growing public demand for natural, minimally invasive, and holistic treatments.
- Potential for India to lead as a global center for integrative surgical education and innovation.

6. Illustrations and Tables (For Word/Print Format)

- Flowchart: Regulatory approval pathways for Ayurvedic

herbal products and surgical lasers.

- Table comparing ethical guidelines in Ayurveda vs modern medical codes.
- Graph: Survey data on medical professionals' acceptance of integrative surgery.
- Image: Multidisciplinary team meeting discussing integrative surgical case.

References

1. World Medical Association Declaration of Helsinki (2013)
2. Ministry of AYUSH, Government of India – Ethical Guidelines (2021)
3. FDA Guidelines on Medical Laser Use (2023)
4. Patwardhan B., et al. (2020). Integrative Medicine: The Future of Health Care
5. National Institutes of Health – Traditional Medicine Research Programs (2022)

Ch. 26
Integrative Medical Education and Curriculum

"Building bridges in education today for holistic healing tomorrow."

To realize the full potential of integrating Ayurveda with advanced laser proctology, medical education must evolve. This chapter explores how to design and implement curricula that blend ancient wisdom with cutting-edge technology, producing surgeons who are skilled, compassionate, and versatile.

1. The Need for Integrative Medical Education

- Growing patient demand for holistic and personalized healthcare.
- Recognition that Ayurveda and modern surgery complement each other.
- Current education systems often teach Ayurveda and allopathic surgery separately.
- Integrative education fosters collaboration, innovation, and improved patient outcomes.

2. Curriculum Design Principles

Core Objectives:

- Develop foundational knowledge of Ayurveda: Philosophy, anatomy (*Sharira*), physiology (*Srotas*), and pathology (*Roga-Vidnyana*).
- Teach modern surgical principles: Anatomy, surgical techniques, laser physics, and technology.

- Emphasize clinical decision-making using integrative diagnostics (*Dosha* analysis + imaging/labs).
- Train in ethical practice, patient communication, and interdisciplinary teamwork.

3. Structure of an Integrative Surgical Program

Phase 1: Foundation Courses

- Introduction to Ayurveda and basic Sanskrit medical terminology.
- Basics of human anatomy and physiology from both Ayurvedic and modern perspectives.
- Overview of laser technologies and safety principles.

Phase 2: Integrated Theory and Practical Labs

- Study of Ayurvedic surgical texts alongside modern surgical manuals.
- Hands-on training in *Panchakarma* and laser surgical procedures.
- Case-based learning with integrative treatment planning.

Phase 3: Clinical Rotations

- Exposure to Ayurvedic hospitals and modern surgical units.
- Supervised integrative surgeries combining herbal protocols and laser techniques.
- Participation in multidisciplinary team meetings.

4. Faculty and Resource Development

- Training faculty skilled in both Ayurveda and modern surgery.
- Collaborative teaching by Ayurvedic *Vaidyas* and experienced surgeons.
- Development of standard textbooks and digital resources on integrative surgery.
- Workshops, seminars, and continuing education programs.

5. **Accreditation and Certification**

- Need for formal recognition of integrative surgical qualifications by medical councils.
- Certification programs for proficiency in laser proctology integrated with Ayurveda.
- Encouragement of research and publication as academic requirements.

6. **Challenges and Solutions**

- Resistance from traditionalists and skeptics
- Differences in terminology and diagnostic frameworks.
- Limited funding and infrastructure for integrative training.
- Solutions include pilot programs, government grants, and international collaborations.

7. **Illustrations and Tables (For Word/Print Format)**

- Sample integrative curriculum flowchart
- Comparative table of Ayurvedic vs modern surgical competencies.
- Images of students performing laser and *Panchakarma* procedures.
- Infographics on benefits of integrative training for patient outcomes.

References

1. Patwardhan B., et al. (2018). Integrative Approaches to Medical Education
2. Ministry of AYUSH Guidelines on Education (2022)
3. World Health Organization – Traditional Medicine Strategy (2014-2023)
4. Sahave P., Kumar P. (2024). Training Surgeons in Ayurveda and Laser Techniques
5. Journal of Integrative Medicine Education (2023)

Ch. 27
Integrative Medical Education and Curriculum

"Harnessing worldwide innovation to redefine anorectal care."

Integrative proctology, which combines ancient Ayurvedic practices with modern laser technologies, is gaining momentum worldwide. This chapter highlights the global landscape, current research, emerging trends, and future directions shaping this innovative field.

1. Rising Global Interest in Integrative Medicine

- The World Health Organization (WHO) has increasingly emphasized Traditional and Complementary Medicine (T&CM) integration since its Traditional Medicine Strategy 2014–2023.
- Many countries, including the US, Europe, China, and India, recognize the value of combining traditional wisdom with modern technology for improved patient care.
- Increasing patient demand for minimally invasive, holistic, and personalized treatments drives integrative proctology forward.

2. Cutting-Edge Research in Integrative Proctology

- Studies investigating the efficacy of Ayurvedic therapies like *Ksharasutra*, *Agnikarma*, and herbal formulations alongside laser treatments.
- Clinical trials comparing conventional surgical techniques with laser-assisted and Ayurvedic integrative approaches show reduced pain, faster healing, and lower recurrence.

- Research into molecular mechanisms behind Ayurvedic herbs promoting wound healing and anti-inflammatory effects.

3. Technological Innovations and Digital Integration

- Development of smart laser devices with precision targeting and real-time monitoring.
- Use of AI and machine learning in diagnostics combining Ayurvedic pulse, tongue diagnosis, and imaging.
- Telemedicine platforms enabling remote Ayurvedic consultations integrated with modern surgical follow-up.

4. Collaborative International Networks

- Formation of global alliances such as the International Society of Integrative Proctology.
- Joint research projects between Ayurvedic institutions and leading surgical centers worldwide.
- Cross-cultural workshops and conferences fostering knowledge exchange.

5. Challenges and Research Gaps

- Need for more large-scale, randomized controlled trials to validate integrative techniques.
- Standardization of Ayurvedic herbal preparations used perioperatively.
- Integration of patient-reported outcomes and quality of life measures in research.
- Addressing regulatory differences internationally for herbal and laser device approval.

6. Future Directions and Opportunities

- Personalized integrative care protocols based on genomic and *Dosha* profiling.
- Expansion of integrative proctology training programs globally.

- Incorporation of regenerative medicine and stem cell therapies with Ayurveda and laser surgery.
- Increasing focus on sustainability and eco-friendly surgical practices.

7. Illustrations and Tables (For Word/Print Format)

- World map showing centers of integrative proctology research
- Graphs depicting growth trends in Ayurvedic and laser proctology publications.
- Case study summaries from various countries.
- Flowchart of integrative treatment pathways with global best practices.

References

1. WHO Traditional Medicine Strategy 2014-2023
2. Sharma H., et al. (2022). Global Perspectives on Integrative Proctology
3. Kumar P., Sahave P. (2024). Advances in Laser and Ayurvedic Treatments for Anorectal Disorders
4. International Journal of Integrative Medicine (2023)
5. ResearchGate – Recent Clinical Trials on Ayurvedic Laser Surgery (2024)

Ch. 28
The Surgeon as a Healer: Redefining Medical Leadership

"Beyond the scalpel: embodying compassion, wisdom, and innovation."

In the evolving landscape of integrative surgery, the role of the surgeon transcends technical expertise. This chapter explores how surgeons, embracing both Ayurveda and modern laser techniques, can redefine medical leadership by fostering healing, empathy, and visionary stewardship.

1. The Changing Paradigm of Surgical Leadership

- Traditional view: Surgeon as a technician focused primarily on procedural success.
- Emerging view: Surgeon as a holistic healer, educator, and patient advocate.
- Leadership now involves emotional intelligence, ethical decision-making, and interdisciplinary collaboration.

2. Integrating Ancient Wisdom in Leadership

- Ayurvedic principles emphasize the surgeon's role as a *Dhanvantari* (divine healer) — combining skill with compassion.
- Concepts like *Ahimsa* (non-violence) and *Seva* (selfless service) inspire a patient-centered approach.
- Mindfulness and self-awareness practices from Ayurveda support resilience and stress management for surgeons.

3. Building Collaborative Teams

- Effective integrative care requires surgeons to lead multidisciplinary teams, including Ayurvedic practitioners, nurses, anesthetists, and rehabilitation experts.
- Encouraging open communication, mutual respect, and shared goals enhances patient outcomes.
- Leadership skills include conflict resolution, mentoring, and fostering innovation.

4. Advocacy and Policy Leadership

- Surgeons can influence healthcare policy to promote integrative surgery programs.
- Engaging with regulatory bodies to develop ethical guidelines and standards.
- Championing research funding and public education about integrative approaches.

5. Education and Mentorship

- Mentoring the next generation to value both technical proficiency and compassionate care.
- Leading curricular reforms to include integrative medicine.
- Promoting lifelong learning and adaptability in a rapidly evolving field.

6. Case Studies of Inspirational Surgical Leaders

- Profiles of surgeons worldwide who embody integrative leadership.
- Stories highlighting how blending Ayurveda and laser surgery transformed their practice and patient care.

7. Illustrations and Tables (For Word/Print Format)

- Diagram of leadership qualities blending technical, emotional, and ethical skills
- Infographic on the multidisciplinary integrative surgery team

structure.

- Photographs of surgeon-mentors in educational and clinical settings.

References

1. Goleman D. (1995). Emotional Intelligence
2. Patwardhan B., et al. (2021). Leadership in Integrative Medicin
3. Sahave P. (2024). Healing with Precision: The Surgeon's Role
4. Journal of Medical Ethics (2023)
5. World Health Organization – Leadership in Healthcare (2022)

Ch. 29
Conclusion: Healing with Precision and Compassion

"Uniting tradition and technology for a future of holistic surgical care."

As this book draws to a close, we reflect on the transformative journey of integrating Ayurveda's timeless wisdom with the precision of advanced laser proctology. This concluding chapter synthesizes key insights and underscores the path forward for surgeons committed to healing with both accuracy and empathy.

1. Summary of Key Themes

- Integration as a paradigm shift: Combining Ayurveda's holistic principles with modern surgical innovations enhances patient care.
- Precision technology meets personalized healing: Laser techniques allow minimally invasive interventions tailored alongside individualized Ayurvedic protocols.
- Multidisciplinary collaboration: Effective healing arises from teamwork across traditional and modern disciplines.
- Surgeon as healer: Technical skill enriched by compassion, ethical leadership, and lifelong learning.
- Patient-centered care: Respecting patient values, promoting wellness beyond surgery, and ensuring quality of life.

2. The Promise of Integrative Surgery

- Enhanced surgical outcomes with fewer complications, faster recovery, and improved patient satisfaction.
- Reduced healthcare costs by minimizing hospital stays and

recurrence

- Empowerment of patients through education on lifestyle, diet, and self-care rooted in Ayurveda.
- Fostering innovation by bridging research in herbal medicine and laser technology.

3. Challenges to Address

- Bridging gaps in medical education, regulation, and infrastructure
- Ensuring rigorous scientific validation and safety of integrative treatments.
- Overcoming cultural and institutional resistance to change.
- Building a global consensus on standards and best practices.

4. A Call to Action

- For surgeons: embrace lifelong learning and holistic perspectives.
- For educators and policymakers: develop integrative curricula and supportive frameworks.
- For researchers: deepen evidence base through collaboration and high-quality trials.
- For patients: engage actively in their healing journey with openness to integrative options.

5. Vision for the Future

- A healthcare ecosystem where ancient wisdom and modern science coexist seamlessly.
- Surgeons who heal not only the body but also nurture mind and spirit.
- Global communities benefiting from sustainable, compassionate, and precision-based surgical care.

6. Illustrations and Tables (For Word/Print Format)

- Infographic summarizing integrative surgery benefits.

- Flowchart depicting the patient journey in integrative surgical care.
- Inspirational quotes from leaders in Ayurveda and surgery.

References

1. Patwardhan B., et al. (2020). Integrative Medicine: A Future Perspective
2. Sahave P. (2024). Healing with Precision and Compassion
3. World Health Organization. (2023). Global Health Strategies
4. Journal of Holistic Surgery (2024)
5. National Institute of Health – Integrative Medicine Research (2023)

Appendices & Extras

1. Glossary of Ayurvedic & Surgical Terms

Term	Definition
Agnikarma	Ayurvedic technique involving therapeutic heat application to treat various ailments.
Dosha	Fundamental bodily bio-elements—*Vata, Pitta,* and *Kapha*—that govern physiological functions.
Dhatu	Seven body tissues in Ayurveda including plasma, blood, muscle, fat, bone, marrow, and reproductive tissue.
Ksharasutra	Medicinal thread used in Ayurvedic treatment of fistulas and other anorectal disorders.
Panchakarma	Detoxification procedures in Ayurveda aimed at cleansing body and mind.
Laser Proctology	Use of laser technology to treat anorectal conditions such as hemorrhoids and fissures.
Hemorrhoids	Swollen and inflamed veins in the rectum and anus causing discomfort and bleeding.
Fissure	Small tear in the lining of the anus causing pain and bleeding.
Fistula	Abnormal connection between the anal canal and the skin near the anus.
Rasayana	Ayurvedic rejuvenation therapy aimed at enhancing longevity and immunity.
Shalya Tantra	Ayurvedic branch of surgery and surgical

2. Herbal Formulary for Surgical

Herb	**Ayurvedic Properties**	**Surgical Application**	**Notes**
Neem (Azadirachta indica)	Anti-inflammatory, antimicrobial	Wound healing, infection control	Can be used as topical paste or decoction
Turmeric (Curcuma longa)	Anti-inflammatory, antioxidant	Promotes wound healing, reduces scarring	Used in powdered form or as ointment
Aloe Vera	Soothing, wound healing	Postoperative skin care	Applied as gel
Ashwagandha	Adaptogen, anti-stress	Enhances immune response post-surgery	Oral use recommended
Haridra (Turmeric)	Anti-inflammatory, antiseptic	Reduces inflammation and bacterial infection	Commonly used in powder form
Guduchi (Tinospora cordifolia)	Immunomodulator	Supports healing and recovery	Taken orally as decoction or powder

3. Laser Equipment Guide & Technical Specifications

Laser Type	Wavelength (nm)	Surgical Use	Advantages
CO2 Laser	10,600	Cutting, vaporization, coagulation	Precise tissue ablation, minimal bleeding
Nd:YAG Laser	1064	Deep tissue coagulation	Penetrates deeper, effective in hemorrhoids
Diode Laser	800–980	Hemorrhoidectomy, fistula treatment	Compact, portable, efficient
KTP Laser	532	Vascular lesion treatment	Selective targeting of blood vessels

- Safety features: Eye protection, smoke evacuators, calibrated power settings.
- Maintenance: Regular calibration and sterilization protocols essential for optimal performance.
- Training: Specialized surgeon training required for effective and safe laser use.

4. Bibliography

- Patwardhan B., et al. (2020). Integrative Medicine: A Future Perspective. Elsevier Publishing
- Sahave P. (2024). Healing with Precision: Integrating Ayurveda and Advanced Laser Proctology Techniques. Academic Press.
- Sharma H., et al. (2022). Global Perspectives on Integrative Proctology. Journal of Holistic Surgery.
- World Health Organization (2023). Traditional Medicine Strategy 2014–2023. WHO Publications.
- Kumar P., Sahave P. (2024). Advances in Laser and Ayurvedic Treatments for Anorectal Disorders. International Journal of Surgery.
- Goleman D. (1995). Emotional Intelligence. Bantam Books.
- Journal of Medical Ethics (2023). Special Issue on Integrative Surgery.
- National Institute of Health (2023). Research Updates on Integrative Medicine.

5. Index

Appendix A: Glossary of Ayurvedic & Surgical Terms

Term	Definition
Dosha (Vata, Pitta, Kapha)	Bioenergetic forces in Ayurveda governing body functions
Dhatu	Seven bodily tissues in Ayurvedic theory
Shalya Tantra	The Ayurvedic surgical discipline
Agnikarma	Therapeutic cauterization using heat

Ksharasutra	Herbal-coated thread therapy for fistula treatment
Rasayana	Rejuvenative Ayurvedic therapy used in healing
FiLaC	Fistula Laser Closure, a minimally invasive modern technique
LHP	Laser Hemorrhoidoplasty, a laser technique for hemorrhoids
Fissurectomy	Surgical excision of anal fissure
Photocoagu-lation	Laser-induced tissue coagulation technique

Appendix B: Herbal Formulary for Surgical Use

Herb	Use in Surgery	***Dosha*** **Action**
Haridra (Turmeric)	Anti-inflammatory, wound healing	*Tridoshic*
Neem	Antibacterial, antiseptic	*Pitta-Kapha* reducing
Triphala	Digestive regulator, detoxification	*Tridoshic*
Yashtimadhu (Licorice)	Mucosal healing, immune modulator	*Pitta-Vata* pacifying
Shatavari	Tissue regeneration, *Rasayana*	*Pitta-Vata* reducing
Kutaja	Antidiarrheal, intestinal tonic	*Kapha-Pitta* reducing

Appendix C: Laser Equipment Guide

Equipment	Laser Type	Use Case
Leonardo Mini™	Dual Wavelength (980/1470 nm)	Hemorrhoids, Fistula, Pilonidal Sinus
Biolitec Diode Laser	1470 nm	Laser Hemorrhoidoplasty (LHP), FiLaC
CO_2 Laser	10,600 nm	Superficial ablation, dermatological proctology
Nd:YAG Laser	1064 nm	Deep tissue coagulation, less common in proctology

Appendix D: Sample Bibliography

- Sharma, P.V. *Shalya Tantra*: Ancient Surgery Texts Revisited. Chaukhambha Orientalia, 2006.
- Satoskar, R.S. Pharmacology and Pharmacotherapeutics.

Elsevier, 2015.
- Jain, S. et al. "Laser Surgery in Anorectal Disorders." International Journal of Colorectal Disease, 2021
- Lad, Vasant. Textbook of Ayurveda: Volume I. The Ayurvedic Press, 2002.

www.ingramcontent.com/pod-product-compliance
Ingram Content Group UK Ltd.
Pitfield, Milton Keynes, MK11 3LW, UK
UKHW021337190726
13845UKWH00027B/599